Advanced Epilation

Sheila Godfrey

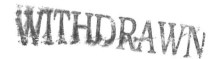

www.heinemann.co.uk
✓ Free online support
✓ Useful weblinks
✓ 24 hour online ordering

01865 888058

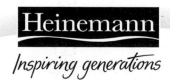
Heinemann
Inspiring generations

Heinemann Educational Publishers
Halley Court, Jordan Hill, Oxford OX2 8EJ
Part of Harcourt Education

Heinemann is the registered trademark of
Harcourt Education Limited

© Sheila Godfrey, 2004

First published 2004

08 07 06 05 04
10 9 8 7 6 5 4 3 2 1

British Library Cataloguing in Publication Data is available
from the British Library on request.

ISBN 0 435 45639 3

Designed by Bridge Creative Services
Typeset by J&L Composition, Filey, North Yorkshire

Printed in the UK by Bath Press

Acknowledgements
Every effort has been made to contact copyright holders of material reproduced in
this book. Any omissions will be rectified in subsequent printings if notice is
given to the publishers.

Tel: 01865 888058 www.heinemann.co.uk

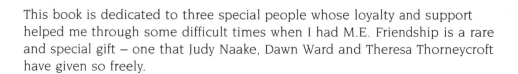

This book is dedicated to three special people whose loyalty and support helped me through some difficult times when I had M.E. Friendship is a rare and special gift – one that Judy Naake, Dawn Ward and Theresa Thorneycroft have given so freely.

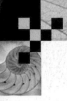

Contents

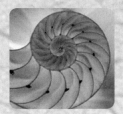

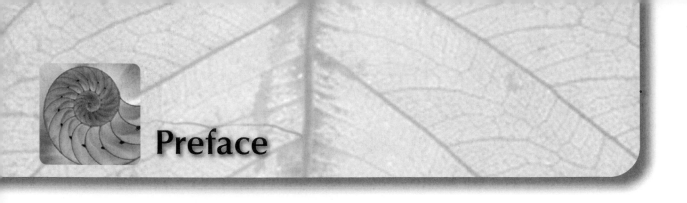

Preface

The purpose of this book is to act as a companion book to *The Principles and Practice of Electrical Epilation*, taking knowledge onto a higher a level and providing up-to-date information on the advanced techniques of epilation for the treatment of conditions such as red veins, spider thread veins and spider naevi to name but a few. This book also gives an overview of alternative methods such as sclerotherapy, intense pulsed light and lasers, showing how they can be used independently or in combination with epilation.

This book is ideal for electrolysists studying advanced epilation for the following associations or awarding bodies:

- ◆ The Institute of Electrolysis
- ◆ British Association of Electrolysists
- ◆ EdExcel
- ◆ CIBTAC (Confederation of International Beauty Therapy and Cosmetology)
- ◆ VTCT
- ◆ ITEC.

During the past few years, the awarding bodies have taken on board the growing need for structured training courses in advanced epilation. Salon owners have realised that in order to meet the needs of their clients they must have electrolysists who are trained in advanced techniques. We have the structured courses but until now not the textbook to go with them.

When treatments are given by experienced and well-trained electrolysists the results are excellent, giving job satisfaction to the electrolysist and a boost in confidence to the client. It is essential that the electrolysist has a minimum of 2 years or 2000 hours post-qualifying experience in epilation for hair removal prior to training in advanced techniques.

Knowledge of the anatomy and physiology of the skin is essential together with a more in-depth understanding of both benign and malignant skin conditions.

This is the first publication to cover the subject in depth. I hope that you gain as much pleasure using this book as I had in writing it. My knowledge in this field was not gained overnight or from one source. My clients, colleagues and students have all made a contribution.

Acknowledgements

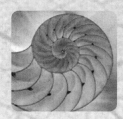

This book could not have been written without the help and input of friends, colleagues and business associates who kindly provided information and photographs.

Special thanks and appreciation go to Dr Patrick Bowler of the Court House Clinic, Brentford, and to Romano Scavo of CTI equipment, Holland, who have both made a major contribution.

Patrick contributed both the text and photographs for Chapter 3: How to Recognise Skin Cancers, as well as providing considerable input for Chapter 12: Sclerotherapy. I would like to record my appreciation for Patrick's willingness and generosity in sharing his knowledge throughout the many years we have known each other.

Romano's enthusiasm for research and development within the Industry is infectious, inspiring me to keep on the ball and up to date with technology. Romano was responsible for introducing me to the benefits of blend for advanced epilation. Over the years I have spent many happy hours absorbing knowledge and exchanging ideas with Dutch colleagues at his training school in Holland.

Thanks also go to Dr Mervyn Patterson of Woodford Medical Services for his contribution to Chapter 13 on sclerotherapy.

Thanks also go to Moira Paulusz, Deputy Editor, *Health and Beauty Salon*, for her encouragement and help; to Janice Brown of House of Famuir; Gill Mann, Joseph Asch of Ballet Needles; Ros Barrett of HSBC Insurance Brokers; Dr Ross Martin, Elizabeth Cartwright, Rita Roberts, Bernadette Harte, Vaughan Daniels and Adrian Myrick of Lumenis, and Jim Stevenson of Laser Hire.

This book would never have been finished without the sterling work, gentle support and firm guidance of Pen Gresford and Janine Robert, together with their team at Heinemann. I could not have done it without you.

Photographs have been supplied by:

Arand Ltd   HEBC
CTI Equipment   House of Famuir
Dr Patrick Bowler   Lumenis
Ellisons   Lynton Lasers
Institute of Electrolysis   Probex.

The skin

Key points

1 The skin is the largest organ of the body.

2 The health and condition of the skin plays an important role in the treatment results.

3 The skin consists of the epidermis, dermis and subcutaneous layers.

4 The dermis has an abundant supply of blood from the **subdermal plexus** and the subpapillary layer.

The skin is the largest organ of the body and has many functions. It serves as a protective, waterproof covering for the body; it aids in the regulation of body temperature and is the principle area of touch.

The health and condition of the skin plays an important role in the successful treatment of **telangiectasia** and **spider naevi** in particular, and also the removal of minor blemishes such as skin tags, papilloma, warts, cysts and moles. Observation of the skin often gives the electrolysist important clues as to the health and lifestyle of the client. This will be covered in more detail in Chapter 6.

Structure of the skin

The skin consists of three main layers: (i) the epidermis, (ii) the dermis, and (iii) the subcutaneous (or subcutis) layer (see Figure 1.1). The epidermis can then be divided into several more layers as illustrated in Figure 1.2.

The epidermis: is the top layer of the skin. It is non-vascular and consists of stratified epithelium. The thickness varies from one area to another; it is thinner on the lips and eyelids, and thicker on the palms of the hands and soles of the feet.

The stratum germinativum: also known as the basal cell layer, is the deepest layer of the epidermis. This layer and the stratum spinosum together are known as the *malpighian layer*, or *stratum malpighi*. The germinativum is closely moulded onto the papillary layer of the dermis below. The cells are keratinocytes, which contain nuclei and are therefore capable of cell division. They are larger than the cells in the upper layers, and are columnar in shape. The contents are soft, opaque and granular. Cells contain melanocytes.

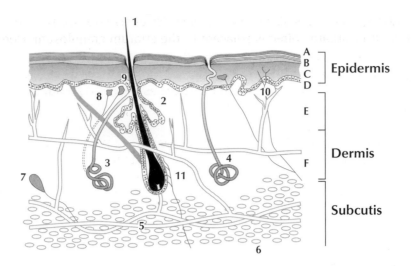

A Stratum corneum ⎤
B Stratum granulosum | Epidermis
C Prickle cell layer |
D Basal cell layer ⎦
E Papillary layer ⎤ Dermis
F Reticular layer ⎦

1 Hair in hair follicle
2 Sebaceous gland
3 Apocrine sweat gland
4 Eccrine sweat gland
5 Blood vessels
6 Fat cells
7 Pacinian corpuscle – pressure/touch
8 Krause bulbs – cold
9 Raffini – heat
10 Free nerve endings – pain
11 Nerve endings to follicle

Figure 1.1
Cross section
of the skin

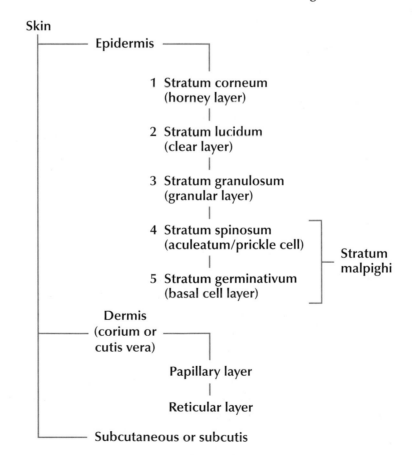

Figure 1.2
Layers of the
skin

The stratum spinosum: is also known as the prickle cell layer (or stratum aculeatum). It is situated directly adjacent to the stratum granulosum. Here the cells are covered with numerous fibrils, which connect the surfaces of the cells. These cells are known as prickle cells. Between the cells are fine intercellular clefts, which allow the passage of lymph corpuscles. Pigment granules may be found here. Cells have flattened slightly.

The stratum granulosum: lies immediately under the stratum lucidum and consists of granular cells. The granules contain a substance known as keratohyaline, which is an intermediate substance in the formation of keratin. Nuclei and other cell contents begin to disappear. The granules consist of a substance called eleidin, which is the intermediate substance in the formation of horn. (See *Gray's Anatomy*, page 1138.)

The stratum lucidum: is present only in the palms of the hands and soles of the feet. It consists of flattened, closely packed cells. Traces of flattened nuclei may be found. The cells are transparent, which allows the passage of sunlight into the deeper layers.

The stratum corneum: also known as the horny layer, is the topmost layer consisting of flattened, keratinised cells, which are horny, hard, and do not contain a nucleus. These outer cells are constantly being shed and replaced from the lower layers. The epidermal ridges interlock with the dermal papillae of the underlying dermis, thereby connecting the epidermis to the dermis.

The dermis

The dermis, containing blood vessels, lymph vessels and nerves, lies immediately below the epidermis. This is the largest layer of the skin and consists of two parts: (i) the upper papillary layer and (ii) the lower reticular layer.

The papillary layer: is situated on the free surface of the epidermal reticular layer and contains a number of small, highly sensitive projections known as papillae. The papillae are composed of very small, closely interlacing bundles of fibrillated tissue. A capillary loop carrying oxyhaemoglobin to other tissues within the dermis is contained within this tissue; tactile corpuscles can be found in some of these papillae. Sensory nerve endings called Meissner corpuscles are situated in highly sensitive areas, e.g. the hands and the feet. The connective tissue is loose and contains fibroblasts, mast cells and macrophages.

The reticular layer: forms the bulk of the dermis and lies immediately below the papillary layer; it consists of irregular dense connective tissue. The majority of the collagen and elastin fibres are found here. The reticular layer gives the skin its strength and elasticity. The epithelial derived structures hair follicles. Sebaceous and sweat glands are contained in this layer.

The dermis is composed of connective tissue, which contains a ground substance or matrix that contains most of the skin's water content in which fibroblasts and mast cells are suspended.

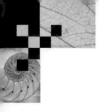

Cells (fibroblasts and mast cells): fibroblasts are spindle-shaped cells which are responsible for the production of collagen and elastin fibres. Mast cells are responsible for the release of histamine and heparin. The function of histamine is to dilate blood vessels, whereas the function of heparin is to prevent blood from clotting. The typical mast cell is large, rounded or spindle shaped with one, or occasionally two, nuclei.

There are three different connective tissues found in the dermis as shown in Figure 1.3.

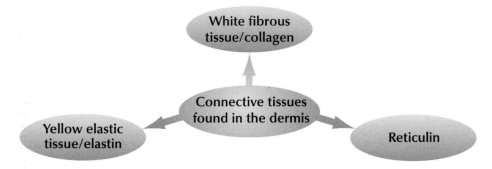

Figure 1.3

Collagen fibres: also known as *white fibrous tissue*, form 75 per cent of the total connective tissue. The fibres are embedded in a ground substance of colloidal gel. Fibroblasts are interspersed between the bundles of collagen. Collagen gives the skin its toughness and resilience.

Elastin: or *yellow fibres*, form 4 per cent of the connective tissue. These fibres run parallel or obliquely to the collagen and enclose the bundles. Elastin also gives skin its elasticity.

Reticulin fibres: are thought to ensure stability between the dermis and the epidermis.

Blood supply to the skin

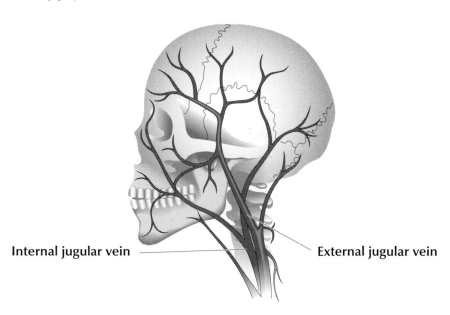

Internal jugular vein ———————— ———————— External jugular vein

Figure 1.4
Veins of the
head

The dermis has an abundant supply of blood from the subdermal plexus and the subpapillary layer. The epidermis receives nourishment from this rich vascular network.

The subdermal plexus: is to be found at the junction of the dermis and subcutaneous layers. This plexus connects freely with the subpapillary layer found in the upper dermis.

The vascular supply to the dermis is derived from *arterioles*, *capillaries* and *veins*. The arterioles lie in the superficial and deep plexuses, and the veins lie in three plexuses known as superficial, middle and deep plexuses. Terminal arterioles ascending into the dermal papillae form capillary loops, which in turn drain into connecting venules.

The superficial and deep plexuses of veins are found next to the corresponding arteriole plexuses. The third plexus of veins is situated in the middle dermis.

A dense capillary network surrounds the sebaceous glands, sudoriferous glands and hair follicles.

The colour of the skin is affected by the amount of blood in the capillary system. When the capillaries contract, the blood supply to the surface is reduced therefore the skin becomes pale. When the blood is passing through the capillaries quickly there is insufficient time for oxygen to be lost so the skin remains a healthy colour. On the other hand, when the dermal circulation is sluggish the blood loses oxygen giving the skin a blue tinge.

The micro-circulation of the skin is responsible for maintaining the exchange of oxygen and carbon dioxide, the nutritional supply to the cells, and for protection from infection by white blood cells and immunoglobulins.

Structures found within the dermis are:

    a. sebaceous glands

    b. sudoriferous (sweat) glands

    c. arrector pili muscles and hair follicles

    d. hair follicles.

Functions of the skin

Secretion

The sebaceous glands are responsible for the production of sebum and its secretion onto the skin's surface via the hair follicle. The role of sebum is to mix with perspiration to form the *acid mantle*, so maintaining the pH balance. Sebum also provides a waterproof film on the epidermis and helps to lubricate hair.

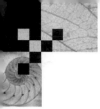

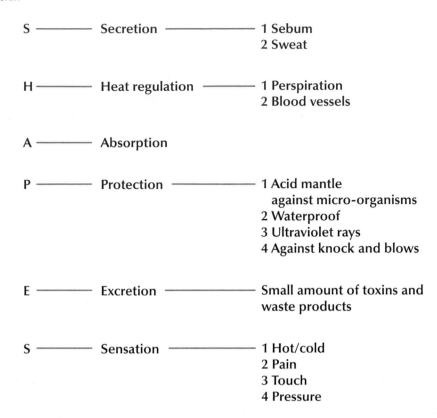

Figure 1.5
Functions of
the skin

Heat (thermo) regulation

The skin has a specific role to play in the body's temperature control. Body temperature is maintained by the constriction or dilation of dermal blood vessels and the evaporation of perspiration on the skin's surface. The skin is capable of containing approximately 4.5 per cent of the total blood volume. When the body temperature is raised, the blood vessels dilate to bring blood closer to the skin's surface. The heat, carried in the blood, is released through the skin. The sudoriferous (approcrine and eccrine) glands increase the excretion of sweat. When the sweat reaches the skin's surface evaporation occurs due to the heat from the blood vessels. This action has a cooling effect thereby reducing the body temperature. Conversely, when the body is cold there is a reduction in sweat production. Blood vessels constrict to keep blood away from the skin's surface and retain heat within the body.

Absorption

The administration of certain drugs, such as Hormone Replacement Therapy, by means of impregnated patches placed directly onto the skin, indicates that the skin is capable of absorbing certain substances.

Protection

The skin protects the body in several ways.

i. Melanocytes, found in the epidermis, produce melanin which helps to protect the skin from the harmful rays of ultraviolet (UV) light.

ii. The acid mantle, a fine film of sebum and sweat found on the surface of the skin. The purpose of the acid mantle is to inhibit the growth of bacteria and prevent the entry of micro-organisms into the skin. The pH scale is measured on a scale of 0–14, with 7 being neutral. The lower the number, the higher the acidity. The normal pH of caucasian skin is between 4.5 and 6. The acid mantle is often destroyed through overenthusiastic use of soaps and harsh detergents.

iii. The subcutaneous layer acts as a buffer, giving protection from knocks and blows.

iv. The keratinised cells in the epidermis prevent the entry of harsh chemicals, bacteria and viruses.

Figure 1.6
The pH scale

Excretion

Small amounts of waste products and toxins are eliminated from the body onto the skin's surface via perspiration. The amount of waste matter increases during times of stress and ill health.

Sensation

The skin is the principle seat of sensation. The papillary layer in the dermis contains an abundant supply of sensory nerve endings which transmit pain, heat, cold, and pressure. The nerve supply also surrounds the hair follicle, arrector pili muscle and sudoriferous glands. Nerves within the skin end either in a corpuscle or free endings. Meissner corpuscles are unique sensory receptors found only in the feet, hands and digits. The free-ending nerves are responsible for the sense of pain. Those nerves ending in corpuscles are grouped into:

- Pacinian – responsible for touch or pressure
- Krause bulbs – responsible for the sensation of cold
- Organs of Rafinni – responsible for the sensation of heat.

Formation of vitamin D

Vitamin D is formed by the action of ultraviolet light on dehydrocholesterol within the skin. Vitamin D aids in the formation and maintenance of healthy bone.

Natural moisturising factor

The function of the **natural moisturising factor** (NMF) is to aid in the prevention of loss of moisture from the epidermis. As the cells within the skin structures move up towards the surface, moisture is pressed out of the cells, which results in each cell being coated with a sticky intercellular glue, thereby holding the stratum corneum together.

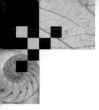

Summary

◆ The skin consists of three main layers: the epidermis, the dermis, and subcutaneous (or subcutis) layers.

◆ The cells of the epidermis are shed regularly and replaced by cells from the lower layers.

◆ The epidermis does not contain blood vessels but derives its nutrition from the vascular structures contained within the dermis.

◆ The epidermis acts as a protective barrier.

◆ The dermis can be subdivided into the: papillary layer and reticular layer.

◆ The dermis contains a rich vascular network of nerve endings, sebaceous glands, sweat glands, hair follicles, elastin, collagen and fibroblasts.

◆ The dermis lies immediately below the epidermis.

◆ The reticular layer of the dermis contains dense connective tissue that gives the skin its strength and elasticity.

◆ There are three different connective tissues found in the dermis. These are: white fibrous tissue/collagen, yellow elastic tissue/elastin, and reticulin.

◆ The micro-circulation of the skin is responsible for maintaining the exchange of oxygen and carbon dioxide, the nutritional supply to the cells, and for protection from infection by white blood cells and immunoglobulins.

◆ Structures found within the dermis are: sebaceous glands, sudoriferous (sweat) glands, arrector pili muscles and hair follicles.

◆ Functions of the skin are: secretion, heat (thermo) regulation, absorption, protection, excretion and sensation.

Review questions

1 Name the layers of the epidermis.

2 Name the layers of the dermis.

3 Describe the skin's blood supply.

4 What are Meissner corpuscles and where are they found?

5 Describe how the skin gains its strength and elasticity.

6 List the functions of the skin.

7 List the substances that influence the skin's colour.

8 Give the composition of connective tissue.

9 State how the skin controls the loss or conservation of body heat.

Dermatology

Chapter 2

Key points

1. The electrolysist is not a dermatologist, therefore 'when in doubt' refer the client on to the medical profession.

2. The electrolysist should be familiar with the basic terminology associated with dermatology.

3. The electrolysist should also be familiar with the symptoms and signs associated with the different skin conditions and the fact that many of these can be present in more than one disorder or disease, e.g. *hyper-pigmentation* post-laser or sun damage leading to melanoma, pityriasis rosea or tinea corporsis.

Clients take it for granted that their electrolysist is the fount of all knowledge relating to a wide range of skin conditions. Not only do they expect her or him to be able to recognise and diagnose their specific skin condition but also to be able to advise on treatment. Clients regularly overlook the fact that electrolysists are not dermatologists! This places a great deal of responsibility on the electrolysist, therefore it is essential that she or he is able to recognise specific skin disorders and diseases. The electrolysist must know when to treat and when to refer the client to a doctor or dermatologist. General terminology relating to dermatology can be found in Chapter 2 of *The Principles and Practice of Electrical Epilation*.

The aim of this chapter is to highlight the specific conditions that may be encountered during the advanced application of electrical epilation, lasers and *intense pulsed light* (IPL) treatments. In Chapter 3, Dr Patrick Bowler covers *benign* and malignant tumours.

Initially, it is essential to become familiar with some of the basic terminology associated with dermatology. The next stage is to become familiar with the symptoms and signs associated with the different skin conditions and the fact that many of these can be present in more than one disorder or disease. This may cause confusion when making a diagnosis, e.g. pityriasis rosea can be confused with tinea corporis (ringworm) when the herald patch first appears, yet the two conditions are entirely different.

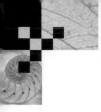

Glossary of terminology associated with skin disorders and diseases

Acanthosis epidermal thickening due to an increase in the number of prickle cells.

Bulla large lesion, more than 2–3 cm in diameter, containing fluid, i.e. blister.

Comedone may be closed or open. This lesion is a collection of sebum, keratinised cells and certain waste substances that accumulate in the entrance of the hair follicle. An open comedone is a blackhead contained within the follicle, whereas a closed comedone, or whitehead, is trapped underneath the skin's surface. Closed comedones do have a small opening on the surface of the skin.

Crust also referred to as a scab, this is an accumulation of dried fluid, serum or pus on the surface of the skin, seen in impetigo.

Ecthyma a pyogenic skin infection characterised by superficial crusting and underlying ulceration.

Ephelis (freckle) a local area of increased melanin.

Excoriation a secondary superficial ulceration which is due to scratching.

Fissure crack in the skin's surface, e.g. chapped lips, which can be painful.

Hyperkeratosis excessive formation of normal keratin for the body site in question.

Keloid overgrowth of scar tissue with a raised, shiny appearance.

Lichenification thickening (acanthosis) of the epidermis resulting in accentuation of normal skin.

Macule flat, small patch of increased pigmentation or discolouration, e.g. a freckle.

Nodule a well-defined, solid lump more than 1 cm in diameter, seen in boils and rodent ulcers.

Papule small, raised elevation on the skin, less than 1 cm in diameter, which may be red in colour, e.g. acne and rosacea.

Plaque a well-defined, disc-shaped elevated area of skin, seen in psoriasis.

Pustule	small, raised elevation of the skin which contains pus, seen in acne and rosacea.
Rhinophyma	excessive hypertrophy of sebaceous glands resulting in an increased volume of soft nasal tissue, a common complication of rosacea.
Scale	visible flakes of skin on the surface of the epidermis, seen in psoriasis.
Scar	appears during the healing process. Skin tissue may be smooth and shiny or form a depression in the surface, e.g. an ice-pick scar seen in acne.
Ulcer	a loss of epidermis (frequently with loss of underlying dermis and subcutis), seen in a rodent ulcer.
Vesicle	small lesion (less than 0.5 cm in diameter) containing fluid, i.e. small blisters seen in herpes simplex, herpes zoster and impetigo.
Wheal	well-defined raised area of cutaneous oedema, white in the centre with a red edge, seen in urticaria.

Changes in skin colour and appearance

Hyperkeratosis: refers to excess keratinisation of cells, or overgrowth of horny cells, e.g. scales and plaques found in psoriasis.

Erythema: general redness of the skin due to temporary or permanent vasodilation.

Hyper-pigmentation: describes an excess or increase in skin pigmentation, e.g. chloasma, lentigo.

Hypo-pigmentation: describes loss of pigmentation, e.g. vitiligo.

Cutaneous cysts

Epidermal cysts: are most commonly found on the head, neck and trunk. They often follow severe acne. They are easily removed by linear incision.

Milia: are keratin cysts located in the superficial dermis. They appear as white to creamy yellow raised papules, either singly or in clusters. The size varies from between 1–3 mm. Many appear to lie superficially in the epidermis, whereas others lie much deeper. They may occur spontaneously or following injury. In some families there is an inherited tendency to develop clusters around the eyes and cheeks. Milia are easily removed through a small incision with a micro-lance.

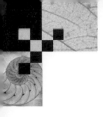

Mesodermal cysts

Skin tags (acrochordons or soft fibromas): are small, soft pendunculated growths between 3–5 mm in length and from 1–3 mm in diameter. They are commonly found around the neck, in the axilla and groin. Occasionally they occur on the upper eyelid or just below the lower eyelid.

Soft fibromas are formed from a thin layer of epidermis surrounding a core of delicate loose collagen. The colour ranges from skin coloured to brown. Soft fibromas are easily removed by cauterisation with short-wave diathermy or blend.

Dermatofibroma: also known as histiocytoma or sclerosing haemangioma, dermatofibroma appear as firm rounded nodules, tightly connected to the epidermis but freely mobile over underlying structures. They are commonly found on the leg and more often in women. Size varies from 0.5–1.5 cm and they may be round or oval in shape. The colour varies from one lesion to another. Some may be pale pink, whereas others may be red, brownish or even creamy white. The cause is not known but it is believed that development can occur as an abnormal response to minor trauma. Dermatofibroma are firm to the touch and are easily removed by excision.

Pyogenic granuloma (granuloma telangectatium): the early lesion begins as a red papule that grows rapidly in size to 0.5 cm or more. As the size increases the lesion develops into a large globular outgrowth, which is bright red in colour due to the increase in capillary vessels. The surface has a shiny appearance. The most common sites are the fingers and other areas that are prone to minor trauma – believed to be the cause of pyogenic granuloma.

Vascular malformations

Haemangiomas: are benign tumours composed of vascular tissue. They appear as a small, raised, red papule which bleeds easily. The cause is unknown but they often appear after vigorous squeezing of skin lesions such as comedones or papules. They are easily removed by short-wave diathermy.

Angiomas: are collections of blood vessels within the dermis and/or subcutaneous tissue. They may be present at birth or develop in later life.

Cherry angiomas (Campbell de Morgan spots): are small papular naevi which are very common during and after middle age. They consist of a group of dilated capillaries. The appearance is of a small, raised, soft, dark, blood spot. The size varies from 1–5 cm in diameter. They are commonly found on the trunk of the body and arms. Cherry angiomas can be treated easily with cauterisation or blend.

Spider naevi (stellate haemangioma): a spider naevus has a central capillary from which fine capillaries radiate that resemble the legs of a spider, hence the name spider naevus. The central body or capillary is often raised and in the majority of cases supplies the blood for the radiating capillaries. Spider naevi can occur spontaneously during pregnancy and if left alone will often disappear without treatment once the pregnancy has ended. In some instances, they may be associated with chronic liver disease. Spider naevi are easily removed by short-wave diathermy or blend. However, some spider naevi are deep seated and respond more quickly to treatment with laser.

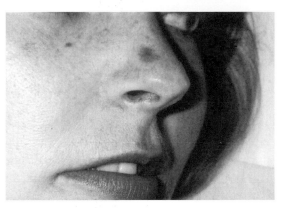

Spider naevus

Telangiectasia: are referred to by a number of names which include thread veins, red veins, broken capillaries and dilated capillaries. Telangiectasia are composed of dilated capillaries in the superficial dermis. They commonly occur on the face, in particular around the nostrils, across the nose and on the cheeks and chin. Facial telangiectasia respond well to treatment with short-wave diathermy, blend, laser and intense pulsed light treatment.

Venulectasia: are larger thread veins that appear blue in colour and are usually found on the legs. They are larger in diameter than telangiectasia and have a tendency to protrude.

There is a difference in structure and appearance between the telangiectasia or spider naevi commonly found on the face, neck, and upper extremities and those found on the legs. Those found on the face and upper extremities are formed from arterioles from which superficial vessels and capillaries radiate, whereas those found on the legs are formed from small veins. Due to the fact that these small veins are subject to the ambulatory venous pressure that develops during a standing position, they do not respond well to treatment by short-wave diathermy.

Treatment of leg telangiectasia with short-wave diathermy or blend is rarely successful as leg telangiectasia often reappear within a few weeks of treatment. The preferred (and most successful) method of treatment is sclerotherapy (see Chapter 12).

Port wine stains: the correct terminology for 'port wine stains' or 'port wine marks' is 'deep capillary naevus'. They occur mainly on the face and neck, arising from capillaries in the deeper and upper dermis. They are often present at birth, varying in colour from pale pink to deep bluish red or purple. The appearance

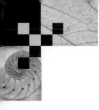

can be improved by the use of some of the newer lasers such as the KTP aura. The process is slow, taking place over many months, and the appearance of the skin can be unsightly during the healing process.

Disorders of the pilosebaceous unit

Acne

Acne vulgaris is a condition that causes much stress and embarrassment in both sexes. Onset is gradual, appearing most frequently at puberty and persisting for some considerable time. Acne vulgaris rarely lasts beyond the age of 30. Salon treatments, whilst not making any claims to cure the condition, do help to keep lesions under control and scarring to a minimum. Exposure to ultraviolet light and sunbeds, in some instances, can help to improve the condition. The condition is often aggravated during the week before menstruation, during times of stress, e.g. examinations, interviews, important occasions, and in humid climates. Areas most affected are the face, neck, chest and back.

Acne vulgaris is due to a defect of the sebaceous glands that leads to the overproduction of sebum. It is primarily androgen-induced and may indicate hypersensitivity of the sebaceous glands to circulating hormones.

Clinical features are the presence of comedones – both open and closed – papules, pustules, cysts, scars and hyperkeratosis of the horny layer. The skin is usually oily due to excess sebum on the epidermis. Ice-pick or keloid scars may also develop in susceptible individuals.

The main factors that contribute to the development of acne lesions are:

1 excess sebum production from the sebaceous glands

2 obstruction of the follicle opening by keratinised cells

3 inflammation as a result of the leakage of contents from the pilosebaceous canal into the surrounding dermis

4 excessive infection of the pilosebaceous ducts through the presence of the P. Acne bacteria.

Rosacea

The cause of rosacea is not known but it usually affects adults of both sexes from the age of 30 onwards, although it is more frequently seen from the age of 45 years. Aggravating factors are heat, hot spicy foods, hot drinks, alcohol, emotional stress, menopause, cold winds and sunlight.

The onset of rosacea is gradual and begins with flushing of the cheeks and nose; telangiectasia become noticeable. The condition may then spread to the centre forehead and chin. As the condition progresses, papules, pustules and scales develop. In advanced cases, rhinophyma may occur, the characteristic signs being hypertrophy of the sebaceous glands and thickening of the skin of the nose.

Acne vulgaris	Rosacea
Develops around the age of puberty, rarely occurring after the age of 30 years	Rarely develops before the age of 30 years
Comedones are usually present	Comedones do not occur
Sites normally affected: the sides of the face, chin, temples, sides of cheeks, shoulders, back, and front of chest	Sites affected: the nose, centre of cheeks, centre of forehead and centre of chin

Table 2.1 Comparison between acne vulgaris and rosacea

Sebaceous cysts

Sebaceous cysts are round, nodular lesions with a smooth, shiny surface, which develop from a sebaceous gland. They are usually found on the face, neck, scalp and back. The cause is unknown. They are situated in the dermis and vary in size from 5–50 mm. The lesion is surrounded by fibrous connective tissue. Cysts contain masses of disintegrating epithelial cells, the contents of which are soft and cheesy.

Folliculitis

This condition presents as pustules and inflammation, which begin in and around the upper part of the hair follicle as a result of staphylococcus infection. Folliculitis is to be found in hairy areas, in particular the male beard, which is often aggravated by shaving.

Pigmentation disorders

Chloasma: is patches of increased pigmentation usually seen on the face during pregnancy. The oral contraceptive pill may also give rise to chloasma. This type of pigmentation usually fades after the pregnancy has ended. It may also occur during the menopause.

Vitiligo: is the name used to describe lack of pigmentation in the skin. Any area can be affected and the size of patches, which may be oval or irregular in shape, can vary from quite small to covering extensive areas. It is most commonly seen on the face and hands. Both sexes of any age group can be affected. The cause is unknown. Patches lacking pigmentation are very sensitive to sunlight and burn easily.

Poikiloderma: is often seen in sun-damaged skin, often affecting women from middle age onwards. Blotchy patches of reddish brown hypo-pigmentation or hyper-pigmentation occur, and in many instances telangiectasia are present on the sides and front of the neck. The skin may also be loose and atrophic.

X-ray treatments and some collagen disorders may also cause poikiloderma to occur.

Dermatitis/eczema

The terms 'eczema' and 'dermatitis' are synonymous, in other words, both terms may be used to describe the same condition. Eczema is derived from the Greek term *ekzein*, meaning to break out or boil over; dermatitis means inflammation of the derma or skin. Both terms relate to a condition that varies from a mild to a chronic inflammatory state. The term 'dermatitis' is preferred by most dermatologists.

Dermatitis may be due to a genetic predisposition, or to internal or external influences. When genetic predisposition is the root cause, it is not unusual to find a history of asthma and/or hay fever in the family.

Clinical signs of dermatitis begin with small, itchy patches of erythema, which may gradually increase in size. Oedema, fissures (cracks), scales and hyperkeratosis are other symptoms associated with this condition. In severe cases, the skin weeps where fissures are present or where the surface has been scratched.

Acute dermatitis: may follow a single exposure to a chemical or irritant. The affected area becomes red (erythema), swollen, and may itch. In some instances, the inflammation will subside and the skin will return to normal after a short period of time. However, the inflammation may increase with the development of vesicles being followed by the formation of crusts.

Chronic dermatitis: skin that is affected by dermatitis for several weeks tends to thicken and develop pigmentation. Scratching of the area tends to aggravate the condition.

Contact dermatitis/eczema: is caused by a primary irritant, which causes a reaction in susceptible individuals. The reaction may occur after a short exposure to an irritant or may build up over a period of time after repeated contact. Substances that cause this type of dermatitis include: acids, alkalis, solvents, cosmetic preparations (in particular perfume and lanolin), detergents, nickel (e.g. earrings and suspenders), household polishes, plus certain house and garden plants (e.g. primulas, tulips, chrysanthemums and celery). Lesions are normally localised to the area of contact.

Phototoxic dermatitis: arises after exposure of a phototoxic substance on the skin to ultraviolet light (sunlight or sunbeds). Phototoxic dermatitis is similar in appearance to sunburn. Pigmentation of the exposed area often occurs, e.g. citrus-based perfumes on the skin, certain herbal remedies such as St John's Wort, and some medications such as Prozac are very photosensitive.

Allergic dermatitis/eczema: is generally more widespread and does not appear immediately after the first exposure to the irritant or allergen. The individual gradually builds up sensitivity to substances such as perfume or certain dairy products. Cow's milk is a common cause of dermatitis/eczema in children. Once sensitivity to an allergen has developed, further contact, even after a period of weeks or months, will result in the recurrence of dermatitis.

The sites most commonly affected are the hands and feet, but any area of the body may react when exposed to the offending substance. As with contact dermatitis, erythema is present and the skin becomes itchy with a build-up of scales. In chronic cases, small blisters, hyperkeratosis and fissures develop. Scratching will aggravate the condition.

Seborrhoeic dermatitis (seborrhoeic eczema): is a mild to chronic inflammatory disease of hairy areas well supplied with sebaceous glands. An increase in sebum production with an alteration in chemical composition may or may not be present. Common sites for this condition are the scalp, the face, axilla, submammary folds and the groin.

The skin may appear to have a grey tinge or be dirty yellow in colour. The onset of the condition is gradual. Clinical signs may show slight redness and scaling of the naso-labial folds, dandruff in the eyebrows and possibly deep-seated pustules affecting the follicles in the beard area of the adult male. When the scalp is affected, greasy scales or dry, scaly plaques will be seen.

Perioral dermatitis: occurs around the mouth and lower face, often as a result of frequent topical application of steroid-based preparations. The affected area develops papules on a pale pink background.

Psoriasis

Psoriasis is a chronic inflammatory condition of the skin. Although the cause is not known, there is no doubt that a genetic factor exists. Any age group can be affected, but it very rarely appears in children under 5 years of age. Psoriasis is aggravated by stress, bacterial throat infection and trauma to the skin, but is improved by exposure to sunlight.

This disorder can be recognised by the development of well-defined red plaques, which vary in size and shape, covered by white or silvery scales. When the scales are removed, the surface underneath will be smooth and red and will show pinpoint bleeding. The edges of plaques are well defined.

Any area of the body may develop psoriasis, but the most commonly affected sites are the extensor surfaces, chest, abdomen, face, elbows, knees and nails.

Pityriasis rosea

Pityriasis rosea begins with the appearance of the herald patch 7–10 days prior to the development of other lesions. The herald patch usually appears on the trunk. This initial lesion presents itself as a scaly patch, with a slightly raised edge, which clears in the centre. At this stage, it is possible to confuse pityriasis rosea with tinea corporis. The disease has no known cause. It can be

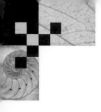

termed self-limiting and usually runs its course within 6–8 weeks. Pityriasis rosea is most commonly seen in children and young adults.

Clinical signs are oval-shaped lesions with well-defined edges and a scaly surface. Macules and papules may also be present. Pityriasis rosea appears mainly on the trunk and very rarely affects the face, hands or feet.

Seborrhoeic warts

Also referred to as senile warts, these warts are not caused by a viral infection and are not related in any way to age. They are normally found on the trunk but may also appear on the face or other areas. Clinical signs indicate hyperkeratosis with increased pigmentation, which varies from one lesion to another. The surface is rough and uneven.

Viral conditions

Warts

Warts appear in several forms. They are well-defined, self-limiting, benign tumours, which vary in size and shape. Warts are caused by infection with the human papilloma virus.

The common wart: is skin coloured or brownish with a smooth or rough surface, which varies in size from a pinhead to the size of a pea. These warts are usually found on the fingers and hands, elbows, knees, and sites of minor trauma.

Plane warts: are found on the face, forehead, back of hands or front of knees. They are smooth in texture with a flat top and frequently brownish in colour. They are most commonly found in children.

The plantar wart: is the size of a pea, or a little larger. These are found on the sole of the foot and may be very painful. This type of wart is also called a verruca.

The filiform wart: hangs down from the skin's surface and may grow up to 6 mm in length. These are quite thick in diameter. The face and neck are the most usual sites for this type of wart. Filiform warts are hard and keritanous.

Summary

The subject of dermatology is extensive. This chapter and the next cover the main conditions that the electrolysist will come into contact with during her or his working life. However, the list is not exhaustive. Several conditions present similar lesions and can be difficult to diagnose, which will affect the choice of treatment, e.g. tinea corporis or pityriasis rosea. It must also be remembered that some skin conditions indicate the presence of a more serious underlying problem, e.g. liver disease, malignancy or polycystic ovary syndrome, which require medical treatment.

Review questions

1 Define the following terms:

   a 'macule'

   b 'pustule'

   c 'vesicle'

   d 'ulcer'

   e 'fissure'

   f 'acanthosis'.

2 State the difference between hyperkeratosis and rhinophyma.

3 Describe the following:

   a milia

   b sebaceous cyst

   c skin tag.

4 What is a pyogenic granuloma?

5 Describe the following:

   a cherry angioma

   b stellate haemangioma.

6 List the differences between telangiectasia and venulectasia.

7 Compare acne vulgaris with rosacea.

8 Compare chloasma and vitiligo.

9 Define the term 'dermatitis'.

10 List six causes of dermatitis.

11 What are seborrhoeic warts?

Chapter 3

How to recognise skin cancers by Dr Patrick Bowler

Key points

1 The incidence of skin cancers as a result of sun exposure has risen dramatically during the past 10 years.

2 Detailed history taking before commencing treatment is of vital importance.

3 Tumours or lesions may be classified as benign, pre-malignant or malignant.

4 When in doubt as to the identification of a skin condition, the client should be referred to their GP or a dermatologist.

One question that is often asked of electrolysists in the course of their daily work is: '*I have noticed this mole on my face recently.*' This is quickly followed by three more questions: '*What do you think? Is it something to worry about? Is it a skin cancer?*' How do you deal with this situation that could have serious implications for both you and your client?

The purpose of this chapter is to give you some guidance in recognising the important features of moles that may be cancerous. However, follow the golden rule which is:

If there is any uncertainty, refer the client to their GP who may in turn seek the opinion of a dermatologist.

So how can therapists do the best for their clients and the reputation of their salon?

History taking

The first step is to take a thorough client history and ask these questions:

◆ How old are you?

◆ When did you first notice the mole?

◆ Has it become enlarged?

- Has it become raised?
- Has it become darker?
- Does it itch?
- Is it ever inflamed?
- Does it bleed?
- Does it heal?
- Does it scab or ooze?
- Do you burn or tan easily? (What is the skin type?)
- How much sun exposure have you had, particularly as a teenager?
- Are you a sun worshipper?
- Have you had any episodes of severe sunburn?
- Do you use sunbeds regularly?
- Have you had any skin problems before?
- Have you seen a skin specialist?
- Do you have lots of moles?
- Have you had any moles removed, were they cancerous?
- Is there any family history of moles or skin cancers?

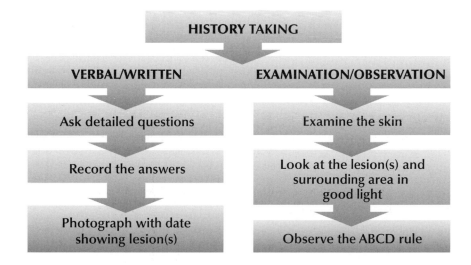

Figure 3.1
History taking

History of change in any way may be a vitally important indicator that the lesion could be cancerous. It may be a new mole or possibly change in an existing mole. Skin types 1 and 2, those with excessive sun exposure, a self or family history of multiple or malignant moles, are all associated with an increased risk of developing skin cancers. So taking a history covering all these elements gives vital clues to the most likely diagnosis.

The second step is to examine the lesion and, most importantly, the rest of the skin. A useful, logical method of assessing a mole is to follow the ABCD rule.

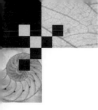

A is for asymmetry. A mole that you cannot divide down the middle into two equal halves should raise your suspicions.

B is for border. A border that is smooth and well defined is likely to be benign. However, an irregular edge that blurs with normal skin may be indicative of a cancer.

C is for colour. The actual colour is not so important as an alteration in colour. A lesion that suddenly becomes darker may be a cause for concern.

D is for diameter. If a mole is greater than 5 mm in diameter, there is a greater possibility of malignancy.

Table 3.1 The ABCD rule

These are just guidelines to enable you to make a methodical and professional assessment. There will always be exceptions to the rule and if there is any doubt whatsoever, then urgent referral could be life saving.

Freckles:	flat, light brown patches of skin that darken in the sun and fade during the winter
Moles or naevi:	are usually dark brown but occasionally flesh coloured. They are most frequently flat, but can sometimes be raised above the surface of the skin. They are oval or circular and range in size from 0.2–1 cm
Atypical or dysplastic naevi:	larger moles with an irregular edge or irregular colour
Malignant melanomas:	pigmented skin lesions, which may arise as new moles or in 50% of cases in pre-existing moles. They arise from melanocytes in the basal and suprabasal layers of the epidermis. As these melanocytic lesions invade vertically through the dermo-epidermal junction, they develop a very serious capacity to spread through the lymphatics and small blood vessel network of the skin. They spread or metastasise throughout the body and can prove fatal if not diagnosed and treated early.

Table 3.2 Useful definitions

These are a series of photographs of various types of moles. Use the ABCD rule to make a provisional diagnosis. A tip: the moles become more serious as the series progresses!

Benign skin lesions

Freckles: a very common disorder of pigmentation. Freckles usually appear by 5 or 6 years of age and are more prominent in the summer. There are racial and hereditary influences; freckles often affect those with blonde or red hair colour. You are allowed freckles in childhood, but those appearing later in life are due to sun damage.

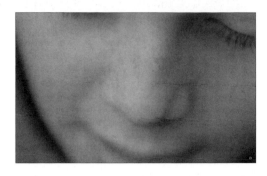

Melanocytic naevi: is the commonest type of naevus and is often referred to as a 'mole'. Over 95 per cent of Caucasians have one or more melanocyctic naevi. They begin to appear during childhood through to early adult life. No new ones appear after this and they disappear in old age. The chance of malignant change is exceedingly small.

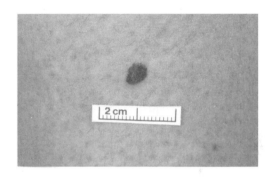

Compound naevi and **hairy compound naevi**: are common benign, fleshy naevus. There is no potential for malignant change.

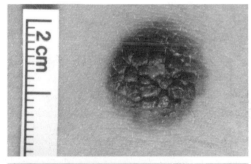

Plane warts: are smaller than common warts and they are slightly elevated with a flat top. Usually multiple, they can cover a large area and can be spread by scratching.

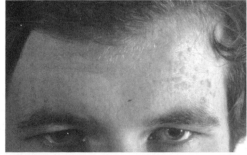

Seborrhoeic keratosis/warts: are very common, first appearing in middle age usually on the trunk and face. Brown, rough and scaly, some can exceed 2 cm in diameter. There is no risk of malignant change so removal is usually for cosmetic purposes.

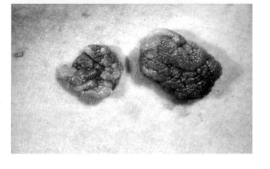

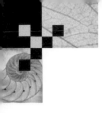
Lentigines: or liver spots are small permanent pigmented lesions usually in Caucasians. Lentigines may appear in the teens and increase through adult life on sun-exposed areas. Laser dermabrasion can reduce their appearance.

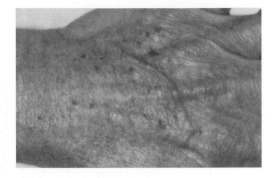

Recognising pre-malignant skin conditions

There are a number of skin conditions that have the potential to become malignant cancers. Recognising these conditions and suggesting referral to a doctor will gain you an extremely grateful client.

Cutaneous horn: can be a marker of malignant change in lower skin layers and is found only in the elderly. Excision and histological examination are advised.

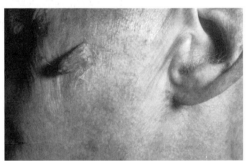

Keratoacanthoma: is a rapidly growing skin tumour, which develops on sun-exposed surfaces of the body. It grows to a size of up to 20 mm within a few weeks and features a central, horny plug. Growth then stops and it may spontaneously resolve over 3 months. However, it is now recognised that keratoacanthoma may be pre-malignant and is therefore best treated by excision with the specimen sent for histological examination.

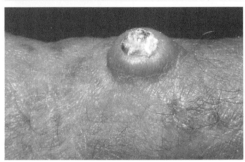

Solar keratosis: are located on the sun-exposed areas of older patients; they present often as red, scaly lesions on the head, forearms and hands. Entirely sun induced, e.g. in Australia 40–50 per cent of people aged over 40 will have some solar keratoses. Cancers arising in these lesions are generally very slow growing. Prevention is the key, but lesions can be excised or frozen.

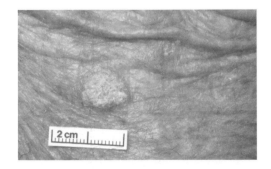

Ctinic cheilitis: appears as grey, scaly areas on the lower lip and corners of the mouth. This condition is the result of chronic irritation from the sun or smoking. Squamous cell carcinoma (SCC) can arise after a long period and tend to be of an aggressive type. Excision is recommended.

Dysplastic naevi: is an inherited trait called Atypical Mole Syndrome with multiple large naevi that carry an increased risk of changing into malignant melanoma. It is important to note the irregularity of shape, size and amount of pigmentation. Regular mole checks with excision of any suspicious lesions are mandatory.

Bowen's disease: presents as a well-defined red, scaly plaque that expands outwards in a circular fashion. It is usually found in the elderly, often on the lower part of the leg. SCC can develop in up to 10 per cent of these lesions. Excision is the treatment of choice.

Recognising malignant skin lesions

Change is the main significant symptom, but sometimes this is a slow process so a high index of suspicion is essential.

Basal cell carcinoma or rodent ulcer: is the commonest, non-melanoma skin cancer with over 40,000 new cases each year in the UK. Mostly seen in the elderly, it appears on the face as a small spot that scabs over and fails to heal. Due to sun exposure, these cancers are very slow growing and only spread locally. There are various types of treatment but excision or radiotherapy is advised.

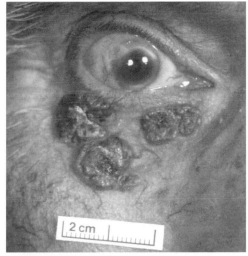

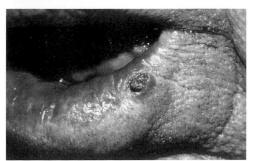

Squamous cell carcinoma: is an altogether more aggressive skin cancer that appears in the over 60s, usually on the sun-exposed areas of the face or hands, and is twice as common in men. Squamous cell carcinoma have the potential to spread and early treatment by excision or radiotherapy offers the best chance of a cure.

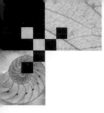

Malignant melanoma: is relatively rare, but the incidence and mortality rates are rising. There are over 4000 new cases each year and approximately 1500 people die from melanoma each year in the UK. Malignant melanoma is more common in women than men, at a ratio of 3:2, and it is the second most common cancer in women aged 20–35 years.

The commonest site for malignant melanoma in women is the leg, and in men it is the back. The outlook for malignant melanoma is dependent on how deep the cancer invades the skin. For example, less than 1 mm equates to 98 per cent surviving 5 years. Over 3 mm, and only 50 per cent can expect to live 5 years. So early diagnosis and excision offer the best cure rates. The treatment of melanoma is always surgical. If there has been general or metastatic spread, the outlook is extremely poor as the disease is usually resistant to chemotherapy and radiotherapy. Recent immunotherapy studies using high doses of Interferon offer a glimmer of hope. Therapists can be the first point of contact or just notice a suspicious lesion whilst performing a treatment. There is great opportunity to recommend referral to a doctor.

Follow-up care is vitally important; keep a regular check on the skin while continually enforcing the concepts of protection and restricted sun exposure.

RISK FACTORS FOR MALIGNANT MELANOMA

- ◆ Presence of freckles and fair skin type means more susceptibility to ultraviolet (UV) light.
- ◆ Presence of 20 or more small benign moles.
- ◆ Presence of one or more dysplastic naevi, so-called Atypical Mole Syndrome (AMS).
- ◆ Previous history of sunburn, particularly in childhood. The evidence for an association between sun exposure and melanoma is based upon large population studies. Melanoma is up to ten times more common in Australia than in the UK. The earlier the age of migration to Australia, the higher the risk of developing melanoma. This suggests that excessive UV exposure in childhood is the most detrimental.
- ◆ Family history of melanoma. Ten per cent of all melanomas are familial, mainly in AMS.
- ◆ Previous melanoma removed.

Types of malignant melanoma

There are several distinct types of malignant melanoma, all are best treated by early excision:

Lentigo maligna: accounts for 15 per cent of melanomas and is most frequently found on the head and neck of older patients. Lentigo maligna presents as a flat, irregular area of pigmentation. Nodules of malignancy can form within the lesion; however, it is very slow growing and can be present for many years. Treatment is by excision or radiotherapy.

Superficial spreading: is the commonest type, comprising 50 per cent of all malignant melanomas.

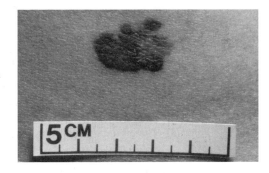

Sub-ungual and acral: comprise 10 per cent of malignant melanomas. They are found under nails and on the soles of the feet. Any pigmented area under a nail should be treated with suspicion and may need expert advice.

Nodular: represent 20–25 per cent of malignant melanomas and are the most aggressive type of melanoma. Raised and lumpy, this type of melanoma also deeply invades the skin and rapidly spreads. This type of malignant melanoma is invariably fatal unless detected early.

With increasing numbers of men and women visiting beauty salons, therapists are in a unique position to give advice on skin lesions. Clients may be anxious and point out a mole that is giving them concern. Others may be unaware of a skin problem and following a careful examination you may be able to give important advice. ***Never, never, be too proud to refer for a second opinion***. Always err on the side of caution and send clients back to their GP for further investigation. Even if the lesion turns out to be benign, your client will remain forever grateful.

Summary

The subject of dermatology is comprehensive and can be a minefield. Electrolysists are not dermatologists; however, they are often the first professional whose opinion the client will ask for. There are many instances when the only positive way to diagnose whether a naevus or mole is malignant is for a biopsy to be taken.

There are three types of moles: benign, pre-malignant and malignant. When in doubt, the electrolysist should, and must, refer the client back to his or her doctor who will in turn refer the client on to a dermatologist. It is essential that prior to giving any treatment a full consultation incorporating a detailed history and examination of the treatment site is undertaken by the electrolysist. This consultation should include thorough questions with written details, an examination of the area, photographs, and, finally, the client's signature confirming that all the information that has been recorded is correct.

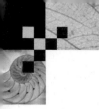

Review questions

1 Give the definition for each of the following:

   a freckle

   b mole

   c malignant melanoma.

2 What is meant by ABCD in connection with the examination of a lesion?

3 What is meant by the terms:

   a 'benign'

   b 'pre-malignant'

   c 'malignant'.

4 List the risk factors relating to malignant melanoma.

5 List the steps to be followed when taking a detailed history prior to treatment.

The cardiovascular system

Key points

1 The electrolysist should know the structure and functions of the cardiovascular system to be able to treat conditions such as telangiectasia and spider naevi, as well as vascular abnormalities such as Campbell de Morgan spots, effectively.

2 Blood is transported around the body via a network of **arteries** and veins by means of the heart, which acts as a pump.

3 The density of capillary networks varies in different areas and is denser in areas such as the dermis.

4 **Perforating veins** connect the superficial veins to the deep veins.

5 There is a difference in structure and appearance between the telangiectasia/spider naevi commonly found on the face, neck, and upper extremities and those found on the legs.

The electrolysist should have a sound understanding of the cardiovascular system in order to be able to treat conditions such as telangiectasia, spider naevi and vascular abnormalities such as Campbell de Morgan spots effectively. This knowledge is also beneficial when clients are concerned about the appearance of small, superficial veins on the legs, or deeper varicose veins. The electrolysist is only able to advise clients on the most suitable method of treatment (which is unlikely to be short-wave diathermy or blend) by knowing the anatomy and physiology of the arteriole/venus supply to the lower extremities.

The circulatory system

The circulatory system can be divided into the:

1 *Blood circulatory system* consisting of :

  a the heart
  b blood vessels: arteries
                       arterioles
                       capillaries
                       venules
                       veins.

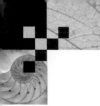

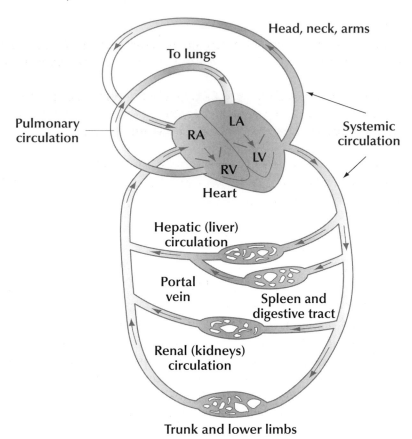

Figure 4.1
The circulatory system

2 *Lymphatic system* consisting of:

  a lymph nodes
  b lymph vessels.

The efficient transport and function of blood within the body is essential in order to maintain health and well-being.

Blood is transported around the body by means of the heart, which acts as a pump, to carry the blood through a series of arteries and veins.

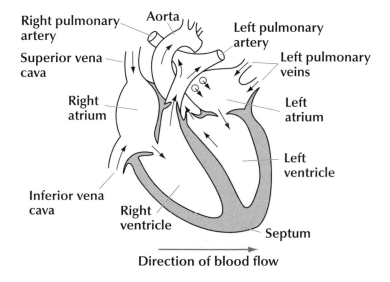

Figure 4.2
The heart

The heart

The heart is a strong, muscular pump formed from three layers of muscular tissue. These are: (i) the pericardium, (ii) the myocardium, and (iii) the endocardium.

The pericardium is separated into two sacs, the outer fibrous sac and the inner serous membrane. Serous fluid is secreted into the space between the inner and outer layers, so allowing smooth movement between the two.

The myocardium is lined by the endocardium – a thin smooth membrane. The myocardium is specialised cardiac muscle which functions continuously and is not under control of the will. The muscle is thickest at the apex and thinner at the base.

The heart is divided into four chambers – two upper and two lower. The septum separates the left side of the heart from the right (see Figure 4.2). The four chambers are known as the right and left ventricle and the right and left atrium. The heart receives dark red, deoxygenated blood into the right atrium from the superior and inferior venae cavae. This blood then passes through the right atrioventricular (tricuspid) valve into the right ventricle. From here, the blood is carried via the two pulmonary arteries to the lungs where the exchange of oxygen and carbon dioxide takes place. Blood is returned from the lungs to the left atrium by the two pulmonary veins. After passing through the left atrioventricular (tricuspid) valve into the left atrium, the blood leaves the heart through the aorta for distribution around the body via the arteries.

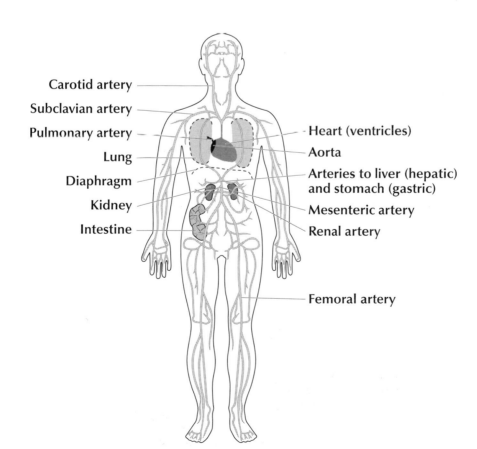

Carotid artery
Subclavian artery
Pulmonary artery
Lung
Diaphragm
Kidney
Intestine

Heart (ventricles)
Aorta
Arteries to liver (hepatic) and stomach (gastric)
Mesenteric artery
Renal artery

Femoral artery

Figure 4.3
The arterial system

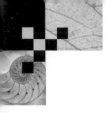

The arterial system

The arterial system is made up of: (i) the pulmonary arterial and (ii) the systemic arterial systems.

The pulmonary arterial system: is formed from the pulmonary artery, which leaves the right ventricle of the heart, emerging at the top where it divides into the right and left pulmonary arteries. These two arteries carry deoxygenated blood to the lungs.

The systemic arterial system: supplies oxygenated blood to the body and is formed from: the aorta, arteries, arterioles, capillaries, venules and veins.

The aorta: carries oxygenated blood to the body tissues. On leaving the left ventricle, the aorta emerges at the top of the heart. The right and left coronary arteries supply the heart muscle and arise at the point where the aorta leaves the left ventricle. The aorta continues anteriorly as the ascending aorta. Its function is to supply oxygenated blood to the main arteries of body.

Arteries: are strong muscular tubes, which carry oxygenated blood, hormones, nutrients and other substances to the capillary network for distribution to the tissue cells. The pulmonary artery is the exception to this rule.

Arteries are composed of three layers: (i) the outer connective tissue layer (tunica adventicia), (ii) the middle muscular layer (tunica media), and (iii) the inner/endothelial layer (tunica intima).

The *outer connective tissue layer* is thinner than the middle layer and is composed of fine and closely felted white connective tissue containing smooth muscle fibres, elastin fibres and some collagen.

The *middle muscular layer* is the thickest of the three and contains transverse arrangements of smooth muscle fibres, which allow the artery to contract in diameter. Elastin and collagen can also be found, with elastin giving this layer its elasticity and collagen its strength.

The *inner layer* is in direct contact with the blood. The inner most part of this layer is lined with the smooth endothelium, which is composed of simple squamous epithelium. The rest of the layer consists of connective tissue and internal elastic membrane.

The function of the arteries is to pump oxygenated blood around the body with the exception of the pulmonary artery, which takes deoxygenated blood from the heart to the lungs.

Due to the pumping action of the heart, blood in the lumen of the artery moves in spurts. Contractile muscular walls also help the circulation of blood between pulses.

Arterioles: (or pre-capillaries) connect arteries to capillaries. The structure is similar to that of arteries but the walls are much thinner. They always have an endothelium and a layer of smooth muscle.

Capillaries: the arterioles gradually reduce in size to form capillaries, minute in size, which can be found in nearly every tissue of the body. Their diameter differs in different parts of the body. Capillaries connect arterioles to venules. The density of capillary networks varies in different areas, being denser in areas such as the dermis. Capillary walls consist of an endothelium composed of cells joined by an interstitial cement-like substance and are continuous with the endothelial cells, which line the arteries and the veins. The capillary walls allow the passage of erythrocytes in single file only. Capillaries permit the exchange of substances between the blood and tissue cells via the tissue fluid. Capillary blood pressure is lower than that of arterioles but higher than that of venules.

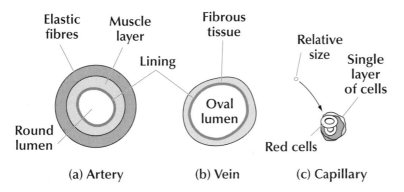

Figure 4.4
Blood vessels, transverse sections

(a) Artery   (b) Vein   (c) Capillary

Venules: are larger in structure than capillaries and form the link between capillaries and veins. It is hard to distinguish the three layers.

The venous system

The venous system can be divided into: (i) pulmonary venous circulation and (ii) venous systemic circulation.

Pulmonary venous circulation: is concerned with returning oxygenated blood from the lungs into the left atrium of the heart by means of the right and left pulmonary veins.

Systemic venous circulation: carries deoxygenated blood back to the heart by means of the deep and superficial veins. Deoxygenated blood is emptied into the right atrium via the inferior and superior venae cavae.

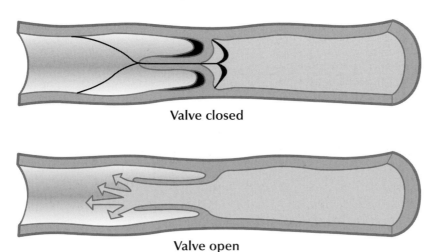

Valve closed

Valve open

Figure 4.5
Cross section of a vein

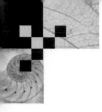

Veins: are similar in structure to arteries except the walls are thinner, less muscular, and they contain valves that prevent the backward flow of blood. Veins are larger in diameter than arteries and also have a larger lumen. The outer layer is made up of thick connective tissue, collagen and elastin. The inner layer is less muscular than that of arteries, with fewer collagen and elastin fibres. The inner layer consists of unconvoluted endothelium with less elastic tissue present.

The semilunar valves found in veins prevent the backward flow of blood and allow the blood to flow smoothly. There is no pulse and blood pressure is low. Skeletal muscle contractions help the deoxygenated blood to return to the heart. When the valves become weak, the walls of the veins lose their elasticity becoming dilated and elongated with fibrous tissue replacing the middle layer. The valves are unable to close properly and therefore cannot prevent the backward flow of blood. When this happens, the veins are known as varicose veins.

There are a number of causes of varicose veins, which include heredity, age, obesity, and standing for long periods of time with little or no muscular contractions.

Deep veins: supply the internal organs and usually run parallel to arteries carrying the same name. The deep veins lie below the muscle fascia.

Superficial veins: lie below the skin, superficially to the muscle fascia, and are often visible to the eye, with the purple/blue colour of deoxygenated haemoglobin blood showing through

Perforating veins: connect the superficial veins to the deep veins. They contain valves to prevent the backward flow of blood during its passage from the superficial to the deep veins.

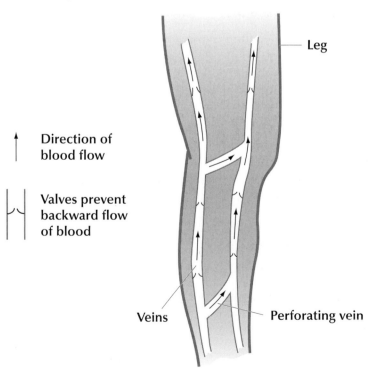

↑ Direction of blood flow

Valves prevent backward flow of blood

Figure 4.6
Veins and perforating vein

The saphenous venous system

During the treatment of telangiectasia to the lower extremities, the electrolysist will need to be aware of the saphenous venous system, its tributaries, and its consequent effect on the success of treatment.

The saphenous venous system is composed of the *long* and *short saphenous veins* and their tributaries: telangiectasias, venulectasias, and **reticular veins**.

Telangiectasia: are small, fine, superficial red veins, 0.2 mm in diameter. They can occur anywhere on the lower extremities.

Venulectasias: are larger than telangiectasia in diameter and have a tendency to protrude. They appear blue in colour.

Reticular veins: are slightly larger in diameter (2–4 mm) than venulectasias and are non-tortuous. These veins are often to be seen 'feeding' a patch of veins. The colour is cyanotic to blue.

There is a difference in structure and appearance between the telangiectasia/ spider naevi commonly found on the face, neck, and upper extremities and those found on the legs. Those found on the face and upper extremities are formed from arterioles from which superficial vessels and capillaries radiate, whereas those on the legs are formed from small veins. Due to the fact that these small veins are subject to the ambulatory venous pressure that develops during a standing position, they do not respond well to treatment by short-wave diathermy.

The composition of blood

Blood is a salty-tasting fluid consisting of plasma and solids. Plasma is an alkaline, straw-coloured substance composed of 91 per cent water, 8 per cent protein and 0.9 per cent salts.

The solids consist of:

1 Platelets or thrombocytes, which play a part in the control of bleeding after an injury and the clotting procedure.
2 Erythrocytes or red cells carrying haemoglobin, which combine with oxygen to form oxyhaemoglobin.
3 Leucocytes or white cells; their function is to ingest bacteria and protect the body against micro-organisms, thereby fighting infection.

The function of blood

The function of blood is to act as a transport medium for the following:

◆ nutrients, tissue salts and enzymes
◆ oxygen
◆ hormones

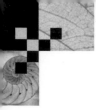
◆ urea

◆ uric acid

◆ carbon dioxide

◆ antibodies

◆ drugs and medication.

Blood is also concerned with the body's temperature control by means of vasoconstriction and vasodilation of the surface capillaries. When too much heat is present the capillaries dilate, so releasing heat to the skin's surface. Conversely, when the body is cold capillaries constrict so taking blood away from the skin's surface thereby containing heat within the body.

Platelets, together with other substances within the blood, are responsible for removing bacteria and micro-organisms from the blood, so helping to fight infection.

The blood clotting mechanism

When the skin is cut or injured blood appears at the surface. After a short period of time, a clot should form over the area to seal the skin, producing a scab. The scab will eventually fall off when the skin underneath has healed.

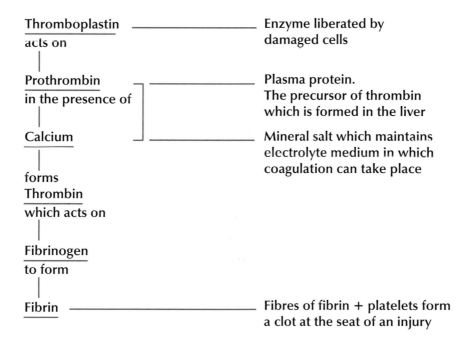

Figure 4.7 Factors necessary to the clotting process

The clotting process is dependant upon a number of factors as shown in Figure 4.7. The health and efficiency of the blood vascular system can be affected by:

1 Badly balanced or incorrect nutrition.

2 Smoking.

3 Anti-coagulant drugs such as warfarin and aspirin.

4 Alcohol.

With clients who smoke regularly, drink large quantities of coffee, or perhaps take an aspirin immediately before the treatment of telangiectasia, you will find that the blood will not coagulate well.

Clients who follow a badly balanced diet that lacks sufficient nutrients and vitamins, or who eat irregularly, may find that the skin is not as healthy and therefore takes longer to heal after treatment. Frequent intake of hot, spicy foods, strong, hot tea or coffee, high consumption of alcohol, or bolting meals down all aggravate the condition and may weaken the surface capillaries.

Summary

The cardiovascular system is formed from the heart, arteries and veins. The heart is a muscular organ that pumps blood through the arteries to the body and receives blood from the veins. Blood returning to the heart is then pumped to the lungs for the release of carbon dioxide and the uptake of oxygen. Oxygenated blood is returned to the heart via the pulmonary veins and the cycle begins again.

Arteries and veins differ in structure and function. Arteries are stronger and more muscular than veins and are responsible for taking blood away from the heart for distribution to different parts of the body. Veins are thinner than arteries and contain valves to prevent the backward flow of blood. Veins return blood to the heart.

Blood vessels are divided into arteries, arterioles, capillaries, venules and veins.

The telangiectasia and spider naevi found in the face, upper extremities and trunk differ in structure from those found in the legs. Facial telangiectasia arise from arterioles and capillaries, whereas those found on the legs develop from small veins.

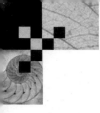

Review questions

1 Describe the differences between arteries and veins.

2 Draw and label a diagram of the heart.

3 Describe the blood clotting mechanism.

4 List four factors which affect the health and efficiency of the blood vascular system.

5 Describe the composition of blood.

6 List the functions of:

   a arteries

   b capillaries

   c veins.

7 Define the following:

   a telangiectasia

   b venulectasia

   c reticular veins.

The nervous system

Key points

1 The nervous system provides a rapid form of communication between the brain and different parts of the body.

2 It consists of two main divisions:

   a *the cerebro-spinal system*

   b *the autonomic/sympathetic nervous system.*

3 Nerves are stimulated to greater activity by heat, massage, electricity and certain chemicals.

4 Nerves are responsible for transmitting messages to bring about a specific response. When sustained, prolonged stimulation is applied, such as during epilation treatment, the nerve begins to tire.

The nervous system provides a rapid form of communication between the brain and different parts of the body. It consists of two main divisions: (i) the cerebro-spinal system and (ii) the autonomic/sympathetic nervous system.

The cerebro-spinal system controls the voluntary muscles and supplies:

◆ the parts of the brain that control consciousness and all mental activities

◆ the nerves that control the skeletal system

◆ the nerves of the specific senses, i.e. sight, sound, taste, smell and touch.

The autonomic/sympathetic nervous system supplies involuntary tissue and controls:

◆ the heart and glands of internal secretion

◆ the blood vessels, causing them to contract and dilate

◆ the viscera, lungs and kidneys.

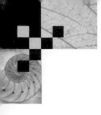

Neurones

Nervous tissue is composed of bundles of very fine nerve fibres, which are made up of nerve cells or neurones.

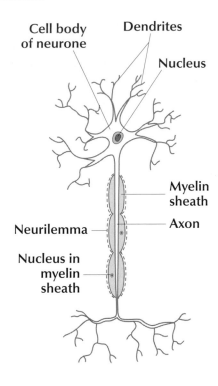

Cell body of neurone

Dendrites

Nucleus

Myelin sheath

Axon

Neurilemma

Nucleus in myelin sheath

Figure 5.1
A neurone

A neurone consists of a cell body containing a central nucleus, granular cytoplasm with mitochondria and a Gogli body. The cytoplasm also contains thin fibres known as neurofibrils. Nissl granules in neurones are formed from endoplasmic reticulum and ribosomes. Extending from the cell body are processes known as *dendrons* and *axons*.

Dendrons and axons extend from the cell body. Dendrons have short branches called dendrites and conduct the nerve impulse inward towards the cell body. One or more dendrons may be present in a single cell. Axons are responsible for transmitting impulses away from the cell body. They are longer than dendrons and are generally surrounded by a myelin sheath. This sheath acts as an insulator in order to prevent the loss of an electrical impulse along the axon. It also helps to increase the speed at which the impulse is conducted. Nodes of ranviers form gaps in the myelin sheath. On the outside of the myelin sheath is a membrane called the neurilemma.

A nerve fibre is composed of an axon and its nerve sheath. Nerves are formed from the axons of a large number of neurons arranged in bundles and covered with a connective tissue sheath.

Properties of nerves

Each nerve cell has different properties of *irritability* and *conductivity*. Nerves that respond to stimulation possess the property of irritability. Those nerves which carry messages to and from a nerve centre possess the property of conductivity.

Nerves are stimulated to greater activity by heat, massage, electricity and certain chemicals. The nerve cords originate in the brain, spinal cord or nerve centres called ganglia. The brain is the largest mass of nerve tissue and the sciatic nerve in the leg is the largest nerve in the body. Nerves are classified as sensory, mixed or motor depending upon their action. Sensory nerves respond to stimulation from pain, heat, touch and cold, whereas motor nerves stimulate muscles to respond either by contraction or movement. Mixed nerves have both sensosry and motor properties. The electrolysist is chiefly concerned with the sensory nerve endings within the skin.

Nerve fatigue

Nerves are responsible for transmitting messages to bring about a specific response. When sustained, prolonged stimulation is applied, such as during epilation treatment, the nerve begins to tire. Consequently, the response to stimulation becomes sluggish and eventually stops.

The effect of epilation treatment on nerve endings

Certain areas such as the upper lip (particularly under the nose) and around the nostrils are well supplied with sensory nerve endings. The upper lip becomes more sensitive nearer to the centre, just under and at the entrance to the nostrils. At the start of an epilation treatment the area can be very sensitive. After a short period of time the continued application of the electrical current, via the needle, causes the nerve endings to tire. These nerve endings cease to respond and the client will find that the discomfort and pain will reduce. The electrolysist will find that, bearing the above point in mind, it is advisable to start treatment at the outer edge of the lip and steadily work towards the centre of the lip. The electrolysist should also work in a specific pattern rather than dotting about from one area to another.

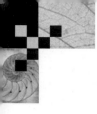

Summary

The nervous system provides a fast method of communication between the brain and the body. It is composed of the cerebro-spinal system and the autonomic/sympathetic systems.

Nerve tissue is composed of bundles of very fine nerve fibres, which are made up of nerve cells or neurones. Nerves are mixed, motor or sensory. Each nerve cell has different properties, namely irritability or conductivity. Those that posses the property of irritability respond to stimulation, whereas those that possess conductivity carry messages to and from the nerve centres. Heat, pain, activity, electricity and certain chemicals stimulate nerves cells.

When stimulation of nerve endings is sustained or prolonged, they become fatigued and fail to respond as effectively to continued stimulation. This point should be kept in mind when giving epilation treatment, particularly when working on hypersensitive areas such as the centre of the upper lip and around the nostril.

Review questions

1   State the function of the nervous system.

2   Name the divisions of the nervous system.

3   What is a neurone?

4   Compare dendrons and axons.

5   Give two properties of nerve cells.

6   Name the three types of nerves.

7   What is meant by the term *'nerve fatigue'*?

Consultation

The consultation provides a golden opportunity to form a link between the client and the electrolysist. In many instances, a great deal of courage is required for the client to make the initial appointment, and further courage is needed for them to walk through the clinic door. The electrolysist's approach at this stage will either encourage or discourage the potential client.

What are clients looking for during the initial consultation with the electrolysist?

Usually, clients are seeking a professional approach that is warm and welcoming – one that is not patronising or flippant, or that makes them feel abnormal or inferior. The client will want to feel that the electrolysist is experienced in advanced techniques and can answer her or his questions fully. In short, the client will want to feel that the electrolysist really does know what she or he is talking about and is competent in the treatment procedure.

Consultation procedure

Client history

A full client history should be taken prior to the commencement of treatment, including a medical history with details of all medication, including herbal remedies (e.g. St John's Wort), noted. See the General Consultation Form a), b) and c) provided at the end of this chapter.

For the benefit of both the client and the electrolysist, it is advisable to give a small patch test during the consultation. This will enable the electrolysist to gauge skin reaction and allow the client to see how the treatment feels. In the

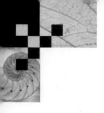

majority of cases, the client is pleasantly surprised at how quick the procedure is and will often comment that the thought of the treatment was far worse than the reality!

Points that should be considered during the initial consultation are:

- the client's skin texture (coarse or fine) and skin sensitivity
- dehydration
- the healing rate of the skin
- the presence of infection
- contra-indications
- the nature and extent of the problem
- the colour of the capillaries (blue or red)
- the density of capillaries
- whether or not the capillaries empty easily
- the speed with which the capillary fills
- the feeder veins – size, position, i.e. entering the nostril, close to the eye, cheeks, neck, etc.
- does the client have an allergy to stainless steel or gold? – this may affect the choice of needle
- the presence of scarring from previous treatment that the client may have received elsewhere
- does the client have a tendency to bruise?

The medical history should include:

- major operations
- blood transfusions
- hepatitis and disorders associated with the liver
- diabetes
- epilepsy
- circulatory disorders (heart problems)
- asthma
- emphysema
- hay fever
- sinusitis
- loss of skin sensation
- constipation.

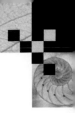

There are a number of other factors that should also be considered carefully. These include:

◆ the client's lifestyle, e.g. outdoor – therefore indicating exposure to the elements and extremes of temperature

◆ the client's dietary pattern – intake of stimulants such as tea, coffee, alcohol or hot spicy foods. Is food eaten quickly, i.e. bolted, or are tea and coffee drunk when they are still very hot?

◆ whether the client has had surgery, e.g. plastic surgery resulting in a few dilated capillaries

◆ the nature of the client's employment, e.g. in hot steamy kitchens

◆ smoking

◆ the frequency and temperature of baths

◆ whether contact lenses are worn. If so, are the lenses soft or hard? – affects blend application.

Why is the above information necessary?

The advantage of taking a full history of both the lifestyle and medical history during the consultation provides the electrolysist with a valuable insight into the cause of the problem, e.g. heredity, surgical, medications such as steroids, extremes of temperature such as cold biting winds, or hot steamy kitchens. In some instances, it may be necessary to communicate with the client's doctor before proceeding with treatment, e.g. circulatory disorders or pacemakers. When the client has an outdoor occupation and is exposed to extreme weather conditions, such as biting winds or long exposure to sunlight, the chances are that without following the correct aftercare the condition will reappear within a very short period of time.

During the consultation contra-indications to treatment may be brought to the electrolysist's notice. When this occurs, a full explanation should be given to the client as to why treatment should not be carried out.

Once the cause of the problem has been ascertained and the condition of the skin assessed, providing there are no contra-indications, a patch test may be carried out. The patch test serves more than one purpose:

1 The client can feel the treatment (which is often less painful than they had anticipated!) before committing to the treatment.

2 The electrolysist can see how the skin reacts to treatment.

3 By watching the skin's reaction, the electrolysist can assess how long a treatment should be and how many treatments will be needed.

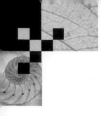

Treatment plan

The consultation offers the electrolysist the opportunity to discuss a suitable treatment plan and the costs involved. The client will need to know how many treatments will be necessary, how often appointments should be booked, and the costs involved.

Many clients are under the impression that immediately after treatment their skin will be clear and free from visible capillaries before they leave the treatment room. Others are under the impression that they can receive treatment 2–3 days before an important business or social engagement and that their skin will look perfectly clear.

Clients should be advised that, in some instances, although rare, the skin may take up to 2 weeks to settle after treatment. This is the ideal time to explain to the client exactly how the skin will look immediately after treatment and over the course of the following 5–7 days.

Procedure for the patch test

1 Immediately before doing a patch test, hand a mirror to the client and show her or him the area that is going to be treated. Ideally, choose a capillary that is noticeable and in an area that is easy for the client to monitor for the skin's reaction and healing time.

2 Cleanse the treatment site and examine the skin more closely using a magnifying lamp. Take photographs at this stage to record details.

3 Carry out the patch test, then examine the skin and assess the skin's reaction.

4 Advise the client on a treatment plan including the spacing, length of treatment, aftercare, healing rate, and treatment stages. Also advise the client of the possibility of scabbing.

The benefits of investing in a good compact camera with super-macro and autofocus facilities cannot be stressed enough. Alternatively, for those who possess a computer, a digital camera will give immediate results that can either be printed or stored on disc. Patience and practice are required to get the photographs you are looking for. However, the rewards are well worth the effort in the long run. Photographs taken at the beginning of the first treatment will be beneficial to both the electrolysist and the client. Clients inevitably forget the extent of the original problem, particularly when treatment takes place over a long period of time. Before and after photographs are also useful for insurance purposes, should the need arise. Accurate records of the dates they were taken, the name of the client and the area photographed should be kept.

After the patch test, inform the client of their skin's reaction and suitability for treatment. Provide the client with verbal aftercare instructions together with written instructions and obtain the client's signature confirming that these instructions have been read, understood and received.

Summary

The consultation provides the initial link between the client and the electrolysist. The electrolysist's approach at this stage will either encourage or discourage the potential client.

What are clients looking for during the initial contact with the electrolysist? Usually, they are seeking a professional approach that is warm and welcoming.

During the consultation, details should be taken of the client's lifestyle, medical background and any possible contra-indications. The treatment procedure, aftercare, skin healing time and appearance should be explained to the client.

The client should then be given a patch test so that she or he may experience how the treatment feels, see the effect on their skin and how long it takes to settle down afterwards.

Review questions

1   State the benefits of the consultation procedure to:
   a   the client
   b   the electrolysist.

2   Describe the consultation procedure.

3   List ten questions that should be asked during a consultation.

4   State the benefits of using a camera for before and after photographs.

5   Explain the reasons for giving a patch test.

6   How long does the skin take to settle down after treatment?

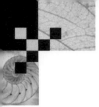

| a | ***The Sheila Godfrey Clinic*** |

General Consultation Form   **Ref:**

Name _____

wishes to be known as _____

Address _____   Contact No. Home _____
_____   Work _____
_____   Mobile _____

Dr _____   Telephone number _____
Surgery _____

Areas of concern:

Hair removal; acne; acne scars; pigmentation marks; skin rejuvenation; facial veins; leg veins; vascular conditions; rosacea; lines and wrinkles; sun damage; milia; uneven skin texture/colour

Other: please state:

Previous treatments:

Skin therapy; glycolic peels; laser; laser resurfacing; cosmetic surgery; Botox; Restylane; Perlane; sclerotherapy; laser hair removal; ear-piercing

Please list any side effects or adverse reactions to previous treatments:

b

Lifestyle:

Diet/eating pattern _____

Alcohol   yes/no   Average units per week _____

Smoker   yes/no   Number per day _____

Sun exposure _____ Outdoor activities _____

Occupation _____   Frequent flyer   yes/no

Sleep pattern _____

Sporting activities/exercise _____

Skincare routine _____

Products currently used _____

Recommended treatments:

Electrolysis; Epilight; MD Formulations; facial therapy; ear-piercing; skin rejuvenation; VL; Laser VL; Photoderm; Erbium Yag; laser resurfacing; Restylane; Perlane; Botox; sclerotherapy

---

To be completed by therapist:

Contra-indications to specific treatments:

C

Name _____ **Consultation date** _____

Address _____

_____ D.O.B._____

Medical History Questionaire

	Yes	No	Details
1. Are you receiving medical treatment at present?			
2. Are you taking any prescribed medication?			List overleaf
3. Are you taking any herbal remedies, e.g. St John's Wort?			
4. Are you allergic to medicines or other substances?			
5. Are you pregnant?			
6. Are you diabetic?			
7. Have you been diagnosed with epilepsy?			
8. Please list any admissions to hospital/surgical operations.			List overleaf
9. Have you ever had rheumatic fever, a heart murmur or any other problem with your heart?			

	Yes	No	Details
10. Have you ever had raised blood pressure, angina, a heart attack or thrombosis?			
12. Have you ever had prolonged bleeding after a tooth extraction?			
13. Have you ever had a problem with local anaesthetic?			
14. Have you ever had any chest problems, e.g. asthma, bronchitis?			
15. Have you ever had any endocrine or hormonal problems?			
16. Do you ever suffer from cold sores?			
17. Do you suffer from varicose veins?			
18. How does your skin heal after injury or surgery?			
19. Are you prone to the development of keloid scars?			

I confirm, to the best of my knowledge, that the above answers are correct and that I have not withheld any information that may be relevant to my treatment. I acknowledge that The Sheila Godfrey Clinic cannot be held responsible for side effects or problems occurring that arise as a result of information that has been withheld. I understand the benefits cannot be guaranteed.

Signed _____

Date _____

Contra-indications

Key points

1 *Contra-indication* can be defined as: 'indication – against (contra)'; in other words, the presence of a condition that indicates that treatment should not be given.

2 *Dysmorphic* refers to a person who will not accept that a particular condition has improved after treatment. As soon as one problem has been resolved, the dysmorphic person will find another that they are convinced has arisen as a result of the original treatment.

3 The electrolysist must not allow herself or himself to be pressurised into giving treatment where it is against the best interests of the client.

Medical conditions contra-indicated to electrical epilation

As stated in the definition in Key point 1, contra-indications indicate that treatment should not be given. A number of medical conditions are contra-indicated to electrical epilation. There are also a number where it advisable to liaise with the client's medical practitioner before proceeding with treatment. Clients should be questioned on the following medical conditions during the consultation.

AIDS: *Acquired Immune Deficiency Syndrome*, caused by the human immune deficiency virus which is easily transmitted via the bloodstream. Evidence has shown that **HIV**, which causes AIDS, is less infectious and more fragile than the hepatitis virus. HIV becomes inactive after a short period of time in the environment.

Allergies: allergic reactions often cause the skin to flush easily. Recurrent erythema puts stress on weakened capillary structures. Consequently, treatment will not be successful unless the main irritant is avoided.

Asthma: is defined as 'a condition characterised by transient narrowing of the smaller airways'. During an asthmatic attack the patient experiences great difficulty in breathing. Asthma may be triggered by anxiety, stress or atmospheric influences such as oilseed rape, flowers and car fumes. Other triggers may be perfume and animal fur. Due to the impaired oxygen supply to the skin, the healing process is slower. The problem will recur in a very short period of time due to the capillary network being weaker.

Bacterial infections: carry the risk of transmitting infection, e.g. impetigo.

Dermographic skin condition: shows an adverse reaction to the needle. Wheals and/or oedema occur where the needle has entered the skin. The healing rate is slower, with the skin taking some time to return to normal.

Dysmorphic/dysmorphophobic: refers to a person who will not accept that a particular condition has improved after treatment. No sooner has one problem been resolved than the dysmorphobic person will find another that they are convinced has arisen as a result of the original treatment.

Emphysema: is a disease that begins with the destruction of air sacs (alveoli). The walls of the air sacs become thin and brittle. This interferes with the lungs' ability to transfer oxygen into the bloodstream and to remove carbon dioxide. The lungs also lose their elasticity. Patients with this condition do not respond well to treatment for telangiectasia. The blood does not coagulate well and the skin's healing ability is impaired.

Epilepsy: due to the precision work relating to the removal of telangiectasia, fibromas etc., it is advisable to avoid giving treatment. This is because the stress of an application of a high frequency and/or galvanic current could interfere with the electrical impulses of the brain. A fit could be brought on in this way. Intense pulse light (IPL) treatment or the bright light of the magnifying lamp could also induce an epileptic fit.

Haemophilia: is contra-indicated to this treatment due to the malfunction of the clotting mechanism.

Hay fever: results in frequent sneezing, which in turn can rupture the superficial capillaries, particularly around the nose.

Hepatitis B and C: are highly infectious and the virus is not destroyed easily. Spider naevi occur in large numbers. Once the condition has been cleared, which takes considerable time, spider naevi may be treated. However, the client must consult with their doctor and obtain the doctor's written agreement before treatment can commence. In this instance, the electrolysist must take extra care to avoid being on the receiving end of a needle stick injury.

Hypertension: nerve endings are highly sensitive. Due to the client's inability to relax, there is a risk of scarring if the client pulls away while the current is flowing.

Keloid scarring: is an overgrowth of skin tissue at the site of an injury. There is a slight possibility that a keloid could develop where the needle has entered the skin.

Liver transplant: due to the risk of infection.

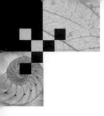
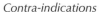

Medication: such as anti-coagulants, e.g. warfarin, prevents the clotting of blood. Clients requiring anti-coagulant drugs usually have a problem with the cardiovascular system. Steroids applied topically often cause thinning of the skin when used for a prolonged period of time. The skin may not respond well to the treatment of capillaries with short-wave diathermy.

Pacemaker: blend treatment should not be given to any client who has been fitted with a pacemaker. Short-wave diathermy should only be given by an experienced electrolysist. It is essential that the electrolysist works closely with the client's specialist throughout the entire procedure. The manufacturer of the pacemaker should also be contacted. When in doubt, the best advice is do not treat.

Pregnancy: naevi, which appear during pregnancy, often disappear a few months after the birth. There is often a tendency for further capillaries to break down during labour. It is therefore advisable to leave any treatment until after the baby's arrival.

Rosacea: is not a contra-indication in the true sense. Although this condition cannot be cleared completely by electrical epilation, the appearance can be improved considerably. Liaison with the client's doctor is advisable prior to treatment. This is a condition that may respond better to treatment with intense pulsed light (IPL).

Loss of skin sensation: inability to sense when the current is too high, which could result in over treatment of the area.

Soft contact lenses: clients should be asked to remove soft contact lenses before the application of blend. The action of the current can cause deterioration of the lenses due to the saline solution they contain.

Viral infections: e.g. herpes simplex, herpes zoster; risk of cross infection.

Summary

There are a number of conditions as shown in the above list that indicate treatment should not be given. The subject of contra-indications should be covered in depth during the consultation procedure. It is the responsibility of the electrolysist to ensure that all the relevant questions have been asked and that the client will benefit from the treatment.

It is not unknown for a client, who presents with a condition that requires liaison with her or his GP before treatment can be given, to insist that she or he has received the same treatment from another salon before without any adverse effects. That may well be the case; however, in order to safeguard the well-being of the client, protect the electrolysist and comply with insurance company requirements, it is essential that the electrolysist does not allow herself or himself to be pressurised into giving treatment. You can guarantee that this will be the one that develops problems!

Review questions

1 Define the term 'contra-indication'.

2 Why are the following conditions termed as contra-indications to advanced epilation techniques:

   a pregnancy

   b hepatitis

   c dermographic skin conditions

   d epilepsy

   e soft contact lenses?

3 What precautions should be taken when a client has had a pacemaker fitted?

4 Why should clients be asked to remove soft contact lenses before treatment when using the blend technique?

5 What is a dysmorphic?

Telangiectasia

Key points

1   Telangiectasia is the medical term for dilated blood vessels.

2   The Greek word *telangiectasia* means end vessel dilation.

3   Telangiectasia occur mainly on the face, particularly the chin, nose and cheeks.

Telangiectasia is the medical term for dilated blood vessels; however, they are commonly referred to by any of the following descriptions: (i) dilated capillaries, (ii) red veins, (iii) broken capillaries, or (iv) thread veins.

Telangiectasia are in fact dilated arterioles, capillaries or venules that occur at the end of the circulatory system. They occur mainly on the face, particularly the chin, nose and cheeks. They can be unsightly and often cause a great deal of embarrassment and loss of confidence to the people who suffer from them. There are a number of causes and aggravating factors.

Causes and aggravating factors

Asthma: due to the transient narrowing of the air passages, the oxygen supply to the skin is impaired. Capillaries with a reddish/blue colour appear on the cheeks and around the nose.

Circulatory disorders: result in weakened capillary walls. Certain medications may aggravate the condition. High blood pressure can also cause telangiectasia.

Comedone extraction: repeated extraction of comedones, particularly around the nose, with too much pressure from fingernails or comedone extractors, often damages the capillaries.

Diabetes: the skin is both sensitive and dry. The blood is slow to coagulate and the skin bruises easily.

Diet: certain foods such as hot curries and spicy foods are very stimulating. Alcohol causes the capillaries to dilate, as do very hot beverages such as tea and coffee. When drinks are too hot, heat from the steam raises the local temperature of the skin. Tea and coffee both contain the stimulant caffeine. Eating food too quickly also encourages the development of telangiectasia.

Pregnancy: spider naevi often occur during pregnancy. If left untreated, these will often disappear within 6 months of the birth. Small, blue veins appearing on the legs during pregnancy do not disappear. Unfortunately, due to the depth of the feeder veins, treatment of the legs by epilation is very rarely successful for any length of time. The preferred method for veins appearing on the legs would be *laser* or *sclerotherapy*. A long strenuous labour can often aggravate existing facial telangiectasia.

Heredity: an hereditary disposition comes high on the list of causes. When questioned, clients often refer only to the mother's history, overlooking the fact that skin problems can be inherited from the father and his predecessors!

Liver diseases: the skin tends to develop spider naevi, telangiectasia and *haemangiomas* in abundance on the trunk of the body. Other areas such as the face and arms can also be affected. The skin bruises easily.

Knocks/heavy blows: such as those caused by bumping into the corner of an office desk, may often cause dilated capillaries to appear.

Medications: the application of steroid-based creams such as Betnovate thin the skin when used over a prolonged period of time or when used too often. Increased redness, skin sensitivity and a tendency to develop telangiectasia are some of the side effects of steroid creams. Antibiotics may cause an increase in spider naevi. Antihistamines dehydrate the skin, which also becomes sensitive to sunlight. Long-term use of Retin A can dilate the facial capillaries through increased blood flow to the skin.

Extremes of temperature: this can include frequent use of the steam bath, saunas and face steamers. Hot baths where the hot tap is left running are also not good for the skin due to the excessive heat. Long hours spent in a hot steamy kitchen have a detrimental effect on facial capillaries. When the skin is subjected to any of the above on a regular basis, weak capillaries lose the ability to dilate and contract efficiently, eventually remaining in a state of constant dilation.

Tight clothing/pop socks: restrict circulation, which puts pressure on the surface capillaries.

Respiratory problems: these include asthma, hay fever and sinus problems. During the height of the hay fever season, constant sneezing tends to rupture the capillary walls. The skin is often sensitive and the client's pain tolerance level falls.

Rosacea: can vary from mild to severe forms. Telangiectasia first appears on the nose and cheeks in a butterfly pattern. As the condition progresses, the skin texture thickens, papules form and the high colour intensifies. The colour can

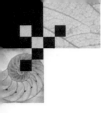

vary from pale pink in the early stages to a deep red with a blue tinge during the later stages. Medical control is usually by the administration of tetracycline.

Sensitivity: to certain foods, harsh cosmetic products, incorrect skincare, and exposure to the extremes of weather conditions. Sensitive skins have a tendency to flush easily. The continual dilation and contraction of capillaries can result in the weakening of the capillary wall.

Spectacles: badly fitting frames and/or heavy glass lenses can put pressure on the bridge of the nose as well as along the upper cheek bones. Unless the cause is rectified, the problem will recur in a very short period of time.

Smoking: reduces the oxygen supply to the skin. Therefore cellular regeneration is decreased and the skin is slower to heal. A smoker's skin often has a grey sluggish, dehydrated appearance. Fine lines can be seen, particularly around the mouth.

Sporting activities: such as horse riding, high-powered speed boats, skiing and water skiing may all result in the development of dilated capillaries. Any sport that involves frequent exposure to the elements, particularly at speed, will have a detrimental effect on the skin. Biting winds will cause windburn, whereas the reflection of ultraviolet rays from snow can result in sunburn.

Sunlight: in moderation has a beneficial effect on the skin. However, overexposure to the sun's rays or the incorrect use of sunbeds causes a number of problems. Tissue fibres are weakened; dehydration of the skin occurs; sunburn and/or prolonged exposure to the sun damages the surface capillaries. Weather affects skin in several ways: cold winds, strong sunlight and extremes of temperature all encourage the development of telangiectasia, especially where the surface capillary network is weak.

Waxing or plucking of eyebrows: overenthusiastic plucking of eyebrows or application of wax on the skin can result in the appearance of telangiectasia. The skin tissue around the eye area is thin and extremely delicate. If the action of removing the wax from the skin is too fast or rough, the delicate tissue around the eye can be stretched and the capillaries within rupture.

There are a number of diseases that can cause telangiectasia and include: scleroderma, erythematosus, rosacea, chronic hepatitis and Reynaud's phenomenon.

Summary

There are a number of conditions that can aggravate or cause telangiectasia. The causes may be hereditary, systemic or mechanical. In some instances, the presence of spider naevi or telangiectasia may be due to disease such as liver damage. When spider naevi or capillaries arise as a result of pregnancy, there is a possibility that they will disappear within a few months of the birth.

Review questions

1 What effect does smoking have on telangiectasia?

2 Describe the skin lesions that appear during rosacea.

3 How do certain sporting activities such as skiing and horse riding contribute to the development of telangiectasia?

4 How do the following medications affect the skin:

   a antihistamines

   b antibiotics

   c Retin A

   d steroids.

The practical application of advanced electrical epilation

Key points

1   Telangiectasia may be treated by: short-wave diathermy, blend epilation, sclerotherapy (legs), intense pulsed light or laser.

2   Facial telangiectasia arise mainly from arteriole capillaries and can be found in the upper layers of the dermis.

3   It is essential that the electrolysist has considerable experience in basic epilation before undertaking training in the advanced techniques of electrical epilation.

4   Telangiectasia needles require a thin tapered point that will pierce the skin easily without causing trauma during entry into the capillary.

5   The use of a super-macro camera to record before and after photographs is recommended.

6   The client should be given very clear and detailed information on how the skin is going to look and respond after treatment.

The presence of small veins and capillaries cause distress to many people. Both sexes are equally affected. Unfortunately for men, it is not possible for these offending capillaries to be covered with make-up! Areas affected are mainly the face, particularly the nose, cheeks, neck, lips, and legs. Spider naevi and Campbell de Morgan spots are also found on the torso.

The treatment of telangiectasia and spider thread veins

Telangiectasia is the correct name for the small red veins which are commonly referred to as dilated capillaries, broken veins, thread veins and split capillaries. Facial telangiectasia arise mainly from arteriole capillaries and can be found in the upper layers of the dermis. Facial telangiectasia are thinner in structure than leg venules and possess lower blood pressure. They may be linear or resemble the appearance of a spider with an enlarged red centre from which fine lines or 'legs' radiate. The latter are known as spider telangiectasia (spider naevi or stellate angioma) and respond well to treatment by short-wave diathermy or blend. The permanent state of dilation makes them easily visible.

The superficial reddish blue veins found on the legs are known as spider thread veins and arise from the deeper venous supply. Spider thread veins on the legs are subject to venous pressure; consequently, they do not respond well to diathermy or blend treatment. Their structure differs from that of facial telangiectasia. (See Chapter 4, page 35). Sclerotherapy is the preferred method of treatment, often reducing these veins by 60–80 per cent. Laser and intense pulsed light also give a 60–80 per cent improvement of these unsightly veins. Whichever area is being treated, in order to achieve successful results it is essential that the root cause of the problem be ascertained.

Treatment of facial telangiectasia by short-wave diathermy or blend can result in either complete removal or a reduction of 60–80 per cent depending on the extent of the problem and the cause. It is never wise to guarantee 100 per cent perfection to clients as they may well be disappointed. The treatment may take several months to complete, therefore it is a good idea to take before and after photographs so that a documented record of progress is kept. When treatment spans many months, clients can often forget the extent of the original problem and may become despondent at the length of time taken to achieve the desired result.

Before undertaking training in the advanced techniques of electrical epilation, it is essential that the electrolysist has considerable experience in basic epilation. The electrolysist needs to have developed a high degree of sensitivity in the hands and fingers to aid insertion into the telangiectasia, a good eye for skin reaction and client sensitivity so that she or he will be able to judge when to stop the treatment, together with the experience and common sense to avoid the temptation to give too much treatment in any one session. The electrolysist must possess the qualities of tact, patience and diplomacy when dealing with impatient clients. **Impatient clients will often attempt to put undue pressure on the electrolysist to shorten the number of sessions by increasing the length of the appointments** (a sure way of finding your way to the solicitor's office and possibly court, or at the very least a disgruntled client!).

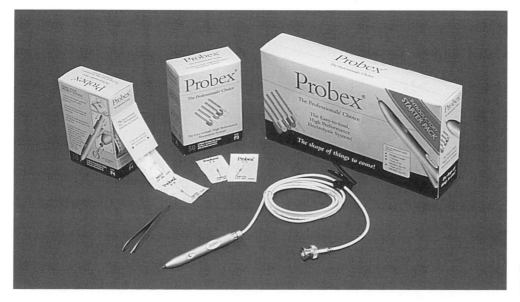

Figure 9.1
Probex needles

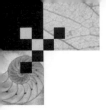

Prior to the commencement of any treatment, the electrolysist should ensure that all documentation has been completed. This includes the client's medical history and 'informed' consent for the electrolysist to treat, signed by the client. In addition, written home care/aftercare instructions should have been given to the client during the consultation. The client should have signed for receipt of these instructions.

Equipment

Before starting treatment some basic equipment is needed:

1   Diathermy or blend machine.
2   Sterile disposable needles.
3   Sharps box for disposal of contaminated needles.
4   Disposable gloves.
5   Mild antiseptic cleansing solution to prepare the skin.
6   Cleanser to remove make-up.
7   Amnitop topical anaesthetic (optional).
8   Cotton wool or medi-swabs.
9   Camera with super-macro facility – an added bonus is a time and date option. For those practitioners with a computer, the best choice would be a digital camera, which can be downloaded directly onto the computer.
10 Trolley.
11 Magnifying lamp.
12 Comfortable treatment couch.
13 Electrolysists stool, preferably with a back support.
14 Aftercare lotion.
15 Aftercare instructions (written or printed for your client's benefit and your protection).

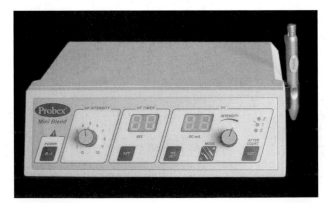

A blend machine

Needles

Before commencing treatment, some thought should be given to the choice of needle. The qualities of a needle used for the removal of telangiectasia and minor skin blemishes differ from those of an epilation needle used for hair removal.

Telangiectasia	Epilation for hair removal
Requires a thin tapered point that will pierce the skin easily without causing trauma during entry into the capillary	Possesses a slightly rounded point that slides easily into the opening hair follicle
Thin and gradually tapered with a sharp point	Possesses a rounded tip
Ideal for easy and gradual penetration to the target depth	Facilitates smooth insertion into a follicle without risk of penetration

Table 9.1 Comparison of electrolysis and telangiectasia needles

Figure 9.2 shows the difference between the point profiles of the two needles. As with all needles, the surface must be highly polished to allow for smooth insertion into the capillaries. A rough surface can cause micro-abrasions and surface capillary damage. Needles are available in stainless steel and gold finishes. Gold is an excellent conductor, therefore the operator may find that current intensity can be reduced.

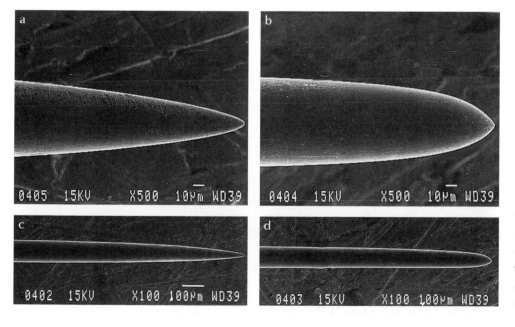

Figure 9.2 Ballet's TEL telangiectasia needle (a, c), compared with a Ballet electrolysis needle (b, d)

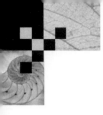

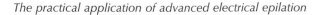

Disposable gloves

In Britain, the decision to wear gloves or not during treatment is entirely up to the electrolysist. However, it is worth remembering that the treatment of telangiectasia is an invasive procedure that entails piercing the capillary wall. There are times when a capillary does not coagulate and blood appears on the skin's surface. Should this occur when the electrolysist is not wearing gloves, there is a very real risk of cross infection with blood borne diseases such as hepatitis and HIV. Gloves also give some protection against needle stick injury.

Use of surface anaesthetic

The application of Amnitop 30 minutes before treatment will numb the nerve endings. However, it must be remembered that Amnitop has the effect of dilating the capillaries. Emla cream can also be applied prior to treatment.

Emla: is a prescription only medicine (**POM**) and therefore must be prescribed by the client's doctor for her or his personal use. Pharmacy controlled medications may not be sold to the client by the therapist. Emla is more effective if a layer of cling film, or similar, is placed on top of the cream. Emla takes 30–60 minutes to become effective as a surface anaesthetic.

Amnitop: is a surface anaesthetic which may be purchased by electrolysists without a prescription. It has the advantage over Emla in that it may be applied to the skin just 30 minutes prior to treatment; neither does the area have to be covered in cling film. Amnitop is a vasodilator; the advantage of this is that the capillaries are more easily defined; however, its use might inhibit coagulation.

The regulations relating to the above surface anaesthetics are covered fully in Chapter 16 page 124.

Camera with super-macro facility

Keeping a record with photographs is a real bonus when clients are beginning to become despondent, particularly when they have forgotten the extent of the initial problem. It is a real boon for boosting their confidence and morale. There are a wide range of sophisticated cameras, with special flashguns and a variety of lenses. For before and after photographs, a compact camera with autofocus, super-macro and date facility is an advantage. Digital cameras provide a golden opportunity for the electrolysist to gain before and after photographs without having to send the film for processing.

Assessment of skin type prior to treatment

The electrolysist should assess the skin type and qualities before commencing treatment. Treatment may need to be adjusted depending on whether the skin is moist, dry, oily or sensitive.

Dry skin: lacking in moisture may hinder smooth insertions due to a build up of dead cells on the surface of the epidermis.

Moist skin: facilitates the insertion of the needle into the capillary; however, the current intensity must be watched very carefully. Due to the high levels of moisture in the skin, the current will rise to the surface quickly resulting in too much heat and increasing the risk of surface burns.

Oily skin: has a tendency to be thicker in structure, therefore insertions will need to be deeper. The pH balance may be disturbed, which in the long term can affect the post-treatment healing rate, particularly if the client does not adhere to the aftercare instructions.

Sensitive skin: responds very quickly to heat and stimulation. With this particular type of skin, there is likely to be a high incidence of telangiectasia present. Treatment sessions will need to be short due to the very rapid onset of erythema. The presence of erythema in the area makes it almost impossible to identify the individual telangiectasia. This skin type is often slow to heal and return to normal after treatment.

Use of aspirin or ice before treatment

Clients are often tempted to take aspirin to reduce pain before their treatment. Aspirin is well known for its anti-coagulant properties, therefore the electrolysist should advise clients against aspirin otherwise the treatment will be unsuccessful. The application of ice prior to treatment causes the capillaries to constrict, making them more difficult to see, which in turn will affect insertions.

The general appearance of skin after treatment

The client should be given very clear and detailed information on how the skin is going to look and respond after treatment. This will often prevent the client from worrying unnecessarily.

The client should be told that when the capillary, spider naevi or telangiectasia is treated it will blanch immediately and disappear in front of the operator's eyes. Erythema will then occur in the area and should gradually fade within the next 2–3 hours. There may be a small raised lump at the site of the needle insertion. A needle inserted into the skin is recognised as a foreign object, this will lead to lymph and subsequent oedema coming into the area. This is a natural reaction, which helps to prevent infection and hasten the healing process. The oedema will subside during the next 24 hours. Some clients *may, or may not*, develop small scabs at the site of the needle insertion, which if left alone will fall off naturally during the course of the next 7 days. These scabs may look similar in appearance to a bramble scratch. During the first 2 weeks after treatment, the treated capillaries may look as if they have come back and may in fact look more noticeable than before – this is a normal reaction that occurs whilst the skin is healing.

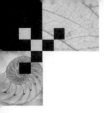

Gradually, the body's elimination system will remove the coagulated matter and the capillaries will fade. When there is an extensive area to be treated over a prolonged period of time, the client may feel that the condition is not improving but in fact looks more noticeable. What is often happening, in this instance, is that, as a result of successful treatment, the remaining capillaries become more noticeable to the client. If the treatment period has been prolonged, the client has often forgotten the extent of the original problem. This is when it is useful to be able to refer to the original photographs.

Aftercare

The spacing of appointments

The client should be advised to return to the clinic after 3–4 weeks to check how the healing of the treatment site is progressing.

Appointments should be spaced at least 4 weeks apart. The skin may look as if it has completely returned to normal on the surface within 2 weeks; however, underlying tissue may still be healing.

Clients may need several treatments to achieve the results they are looking for. The majority of clients will listen to the advice of their electrolysist, although others will be impatient to complete the treatment. This could mean that the electrolysist is pressurised by the client into giving longer treatments than is advisable or booking sessions too frequently.

Aftercare instructions

Strict adherence to aftercare instructions is vital for the achievement of successful results. These should be explained very carefully to the client to ensure that they are understood. This should then be followed with written instructions so that no misunderstandings arise.

The following points comprise essential aftercare instructions.

1 A clear description of the skin's appearance should be given to the client. She or he should be made aware of the changes that will occur over the next few days.

2 Clients should be advised not to touch the treatment area to avoid the risk of post-treatment infection.

3 Clients should be instructed not to stretch the treatment site. Stretching the skin after treatment could reopen the capillary.

4 The use of aftercare lotion or cream (according to the electrolysist's preference) should be explained to the client together with the role of aftercare preparations and the frequency of use.

5 Make-up should not be applied to the area for 24 hours. After that time, it is advisable for the client to apply her aftercare lotion or cream underneath her make-up to provide additional protection.

6   Give very clear and concise instructions relating to the use and application of the chosen aftercare lotion or cream.

7   Clients should be told that any scabs that may form will take the appearance of a mild bramble scratch and will fall off naturally over the course of a few days. *These scabs must not be picked off* but allowed to drop off naturally. When scabs are picked off there is a risk of opening up the site of the treatment, which consequently increases the possibility of post-treatment infection.

8   When the sides of the nostrils have been treated, or the bridge of the nose, clients should be advised against vigorous blowing of the nose for several days.

9   Energetic exercise should not be taken for at least 48 hours after treatment. Exercise will increase general and local blood circulation, which should be avoided for a short period of time to allow the skin to commence healing and prevent the clot in the treated capillaries from being dislodged.

10   Clients should be advised against exposure to sunlight, both natural and artificial, for 48 hours. Heat on heat increases the incidence of post-treatment hyper-pigmentation. The use of suitable sunblock preparations should be recommended.

11   Swimming should be avoided for 48 hours. The chemicals in the water can irritate the skin. It is not unknown for infections to be picked up at the local swimming baths.

In the unlikely event that a problem may arise or the client is worried

She or he should be advised to contact the electrolysist who should be able to put the client's mind at rest. However, this very rarely happens when the aftercare instructions have been explained in full.

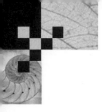

Summary

The treatment of telangiectasia by blend and short-wave diathermy works well in the majority of cases. However, it is advisable to ensure that clients' expectations are realistic. By indicating to clients that a 60–80 per cent improvement is realistic they will not expect every single capillary to vanish. Instances where a higher percentage is achieved can be seen as a bonus.

Needles specifically designed for the treatment of telangiectasia are now available. These have a much sharper, more pointed end than those used for hair removal. This permits easy entry of the needle into the capillary without damaging the skin.

The electrolysist should always wear protective gloves when treating telangiectasia due to the fact that the needle is coming into direct contact with blood during the treatment.

Detailed verbal aftercare directions should be given to all clients immediately after treatment. Ideally, the written home care instructions should be discussed during the consultation and a copy given to the client to take home. The treatment consent form and receipt for written aftercare details should be signed prior to treatment.

The electrolysist, as the trained professional, should control the number, and frequency of treatments, as well as the duration and current intensity. **Under no circumstances should the electrolysist allow herself/himself to be pressurised into taking shortcuts by the client**.

Review questions

1 Define the term 'telangiectasia'.

2 List the areas of the body where telangiectasia are most commonly found.

3 List the equipment that is used during advanced electrical epilation.

4 List the benefits of taking 'before and after' photographs.

5 Explain why the electrolysist should wear disposable gloves when giving treatment.

6 Describe how the client's specific skin type can affect treatment.

7 Explain why the client should be advised against taking aspirin or applying ice to the skin prior to treatment.

8 State the aftercare advice that should be given to clients.

9 Why should the client be asked to sign:

   a a consent form before treatment

   b a receipt for home care/aftercare instructions.

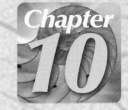

Short-wave diathermy

Short-wave diathermy has been the most popular method of treatment for facial telangiectasia, Campbell de Morgan spots, spider naevi and skin tags for many years. When applied correctly by skilled electrolysists, the results are excellent. Short-wave diathermy has proved to be less effective when treating spider leg veins, which respond better to sclerotherapy, or in some instances laser and intense pulsed light.

The treatment of telangiectasia

The treatment of telangiectasia is a very rewarding treatment to do as the electrolysist can see the results almost immediately. The capillaries disappear as the current flows. A thorough consultation and patch test is essential before starting treatment.

Treatment steps

1   The area should be cleansed thoroughly before treatment to remove any traces of make-up, then wiped over with medi-wipes, weak hibitaine solution, tea tree solution or similar to ensure that the area is free from traces of cream, oil, germs and bacteria. It is not advisable to use surgical spirit, which is extremely drying to the skin.

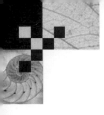

2　A topical anaesthetic cream, such as Amnitop, may be applied to the treatment site 30 minutes before the treatment. Emla cream should be applied much earlier, according to the doctor's instructions, and is a prescription only preparation.

3　The next step is to select the needle and open the packet in front of the client, unless the client has a phobia of needles.

4　Establish the feeder capillary by gently stroking along its length, watching very carefully to see where the vein is filling from. This will show the direction of blood flow in the capillaries. The aim of the treatment is to form a blood clot in the capillary to stop the flow of blood whilst at the same time coagulating the capillary walls. Alternatively, press a finger onto the middle of the capillary. The capillary will empty; it will then be possible to observe the direction of the blood flow as the capillary refills.

5　Turn on the high frequency/short-wave diathermy intensity. The intensity setting will vary according to the machine being used. The current intensity used during the treatment of telangiectasia will be much lower than that used for hair removal.

6　Gently insert the needle into the capillary or vein. Depress the finger-switch or foot pedal and allow the current to flow gently until the capillary or vein blanches and the capillary looks as if it has disappeared. The action of high frequency current in this treatment is two-fold:

a　a coagulated clot forms
b　evaporation of moisture at the needle point.

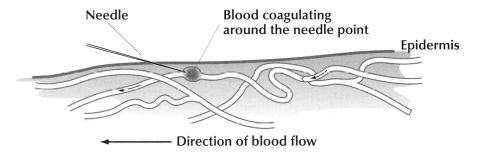

Figure 10.1
Needle insertion

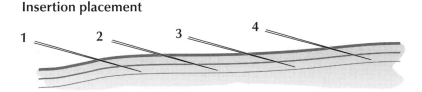

Figure 10.2
Insertion placement

Allow sufficient healing gaps in between insertions when treating linear veins

7　With slightly longer or larger veins, it may be necessary to make several insertions along the vein. Sufficient space must be left in between insertions to allow a healing gap and prevent the skin from overheating.

8   Switch off the current and gently remove the needle, taking care not to
    dislodge the blood clot otherwise the capillary will start to bleed. When
    the high frequency intensity is too high, the coagulated blood will often
    stick to the needle and become dislodged when the needle is removed
    from the skin. The treated capillary or vein will then bleed and the
    treatment will not be successful.

9   Do not be tempted to treat every vein, but be sure to leave sufficient
    space in between capillaries. This will prevent excess build-up of heat.
    When too much treatment is applied to a small area the skin overheats,
    consequently taking much longer to heal. Long-term damage may also
    result from over treatment. During treatment the electrolysist should
    watch the skin reaction and the client's pain tolerance level carefully,
    and should note changes throughout.

10 After completion of the treatment, apply aftercare. The chosen aftercare
    should be soothing, protect against the entry of germs or infection,
    promote the healing of the skin, and ideally provide camouflage to the
    area. The client should be given written aftercare instructions and advice
    regarding the application of aftercare cream or lotion. Detailed aftercare
    instructions are given in Chapter 9.

The treatment of spider naevi

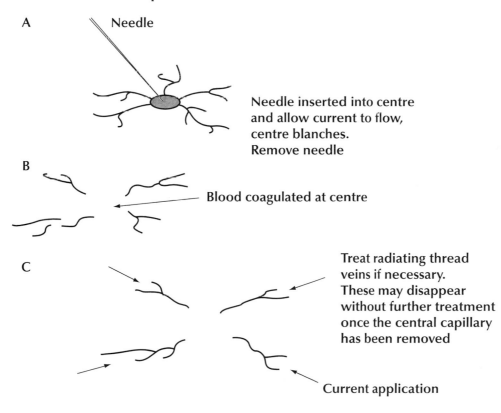

Figure 10.3 Needle insertion for the treatment of spider naevus

The central body of the spider naevus is the main target for treatment. In many
instances, once the centre of the naevus has been treated, the radiating
telangiectasia are deprived of their blood supply and will disappear without
further treatment.

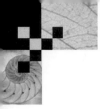

Treatment steps

1 Follow the first three steps of the procedure for the treatment of telangiectasia.

2 Establish the direction of the blood flow by pressing on the main body of the naevus, the blood will then disappear. Watch carefully to see whether the naevus fills from the centre or whether the blood returns via the radiating capillaries. The naevus normally fills from the central capillary.

3 Select the needle size according to the size of the naevus. The most commonly used sizes are Tel 3 and Tel 4.

4 Set the high frequency current a little higher than when treating thread telangiectasia and gently insert the needle into the central body of the naevus.

5 Allow the current to flow until the naevus blanches. It may be necessary to make several insertions into larger spider naevi. Care must be taken to avoid applying too much heat to the area.

6 Once coagulation has taken place, stop the current flow and gently withdraw the needle without dislodging the clot. Should the clot become dislodged, the capillary may start to bleed. However, to avoid over treatment, the application of further high frequency current to seal the capillary again must *not* be given at this time.

7 A small crust or scab often appears over the treatment site. It is important that this is not picked off but allowed to fall off naturally within a few days.

8 Apply aftercare.

The treatment technique for Campbell de Morgan spots

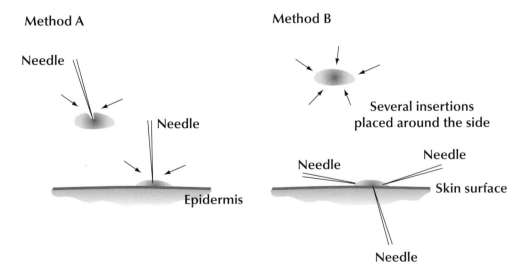

Figure 10.4 Needle insertion for the treatment of Campbell de Morgan spots

These small papular naevi (also known as cherry angioma) are very common during and after middle age, usually on the chest and back. They consist of a group of dilated capillaries, which look like a small, raised, soft, dark, blood spot. The size varies from 1–5 mm in diameter.

It is not necessary to find the direction of blood flow entering these lesions. Treatment is adjusted to treat individual capillaries by inserting around the side of the angioma and allowing the current to flow. Several insertions may be required. The needle size will depend on the size of the angioma. The current should be allowed to flow until the colour of the blood becomes darker or disappears. Angiomas that are larger than 4 mm should be treated in two or more treatments. When coagulation takes place, the angioma will shrink, leaving a flat surface. Crusts will form and should drop off naturally within 7–10 days. They should never be picked off.

The removal of skin tags

Skin tags (acrochordons or soft fibromas) are small, soft pendunculated growths between 3–5 mm in length and from 1–3 mm in diameter. They are commonly found around the neck, in the axilla and groin, and are easily removed with short-wave diathermy.

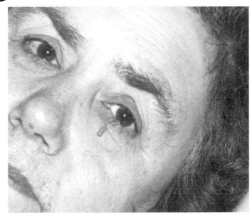

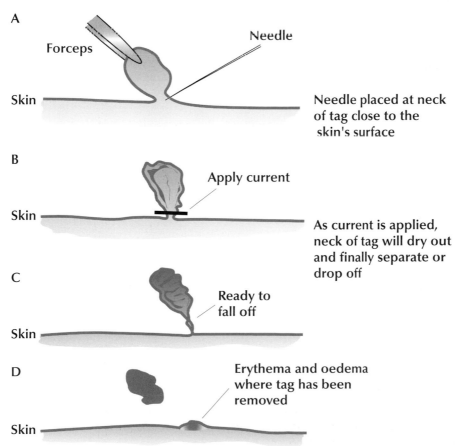

A

Forceps

Needle

Skin

Needle placed at neck of tag close to the skin's surface

B

Apply current

Skin

As current is applied, neck of tag will dry out and finally separate or drop off

C

Ready to fall off

Skin

D

Erythema and oedema where tag has been removed

Skin

Figure 10.5
Removal of skin tags

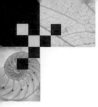

Treatment steps

1 Select the needle size according to the size of the skin tag.

2 Set the current to a higher intensity than that used for the treatment of telangiectasia. The aim when removing skin tags is to cauterise the tag at the junction with the epidermis.

3 Gently hold the tag with tweezers, lifting it away from the skin's surface.

4 Stroke the needle along the neck of the tag, gradually cauterising the neck of the tag until it separates from the skin.

5 The tag will separate cleanly from the skin just leaving an area of oedema and erythema. This may take 48 hours to settle down. A crust or scab may then appear and will fall off within a few days or up to 2 weeks.

6 In some instances the skin tag dries out during treatment, leaving a small dark or black strand of dried skin. This can be left to fall off in the course of the following few days.

7 Apply aftercare.

The skin's appearance after treatment with short-wave diathermy

Initially, there will be general erythema in the area; this should disappear within a short period of time. Small raised lumps may appear at the site of needle insertion; these should gradually disappear during the next day or so following treatment. Small bramble-like scabs may be present for up to 7 days and should fall off naturally.

The causes of scarring due to short-wave diathermy

There are several ways in which scars can occur as a result of treatment.

1 Incorrect hygiene prior to, during or after treatment. There has been a noticeable reduction in claims arising as a result of infection since the advent of pre-sterilised disposable needles.

2 The needle has been inserted too deeply into the skin, missing the capillary and destroying skin tissue lying below. White marks (hypo-pigmentation) will be present and may not fade with time. Pit marks or depressions will be visible.

3 The current intensity is too high, burning the surface of the skin and the layers below. Brown pigment marks will appear when too much heat has been used (hyper-pigmentation).

4 Tenting of the skin due to too high a current will cause the skin to stick to the needle and pull when the needle is removed. Scabs will form and pit marks or depressions may form underneath.

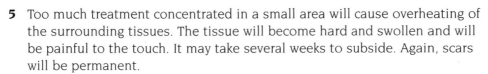

5 Too much treatment concentrated in a small area will cause overheating of the surrounding tissues. The tissue will become hard and swollen and will be painful to the touch. It may take several weeks to subside. Again, scars will be permanent.

6 Too long a treatment session will result in a build up of heat in the surrounding tissues with the same result as detailed in point 5.

7 Scarring, hypo-pigmentation or hyper-pigmentation can occur when the client does not follow the aftercare procedures. This may be due to infection occurring as a result of the client fingering the area, applying make-up too soon after treatment, or picking up an infection in the swimming pool. Brown pigmentation marks will become noticeable after overexposure to heat as a result of sunbathing or using a sunbed.

Summary

The application of short-wave diathermy to treat telangiectasia, Campbell de Morgan spots and spider naevi is very effective. The technique needs to be adjusted according to the specific condition being treated, e.g. facial linear telangiectasia are treated by allowing the current to flow along the length of the capillary with the needle being inserted at the end of the capillary, whereas the treatment of spider naevi involves the central body being treated first.

Treatment sessions should be booked at least 4 weeks apart to prevent over treatment of the area. The telangiectasia disappears during the treatment but gradually reappears shortly afterwards. They appear darker in colour, often looking worse than they did before treatment. Gradually these will fade and within 3–4 weeks the treated capillaries will fade.

Small scabs may, or may not, form where the needle has been inserted into the skin. These will look like small bramble scratches and will fall off naturally within a short period of time.

The skin can be left with scars if the treatment is not applied correctly or if the client fails to follow the home care instructions. When the treatment is carried out correctly and the home care instructions have been followed carefully, the results will be good.

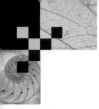

Review questions

1 Explain the benefits of using preparations such as Amnitop and Emla cream prior to treatment.

2 Why is it important to establish which are the 'feeder veins' before commencing treatment?

3 Define the 'aim' when treating capillaries with short-wave diathermy.

4 Describe the appearance of the skin when too much treatment has been given in a concentrated area.

5 Describe the skin's appearance:

   a immediately after treatment

   b 2–7 days later.

6 List five ways in which the skin can be left with scars after treatment.

7 Define 'tenting of the skin'.

8 Define:

   a hypo-pigmentation

   b hyper-pigmentation.

Treatment with blend

Chapter 11

Key points

1 The blended action of galvanic and short-wave diathermy currents gives a gentler treatment to the skin.

2 Galvanic current is used to gently dissolve the skin when the needle is inserted.

3 High frequency coagulates the blood to form a clot.

4 The application of cataphoresis after treatment helps to reduce localised swelling and encourages vasoconstriction.

5 A small amount of galvanic current is used to slightly dissolve the clot around the needle when the needle is withdrawn. This prevents the clot from being dislodged when the needle is removed.

The blend of galvanic and high frequency currents during the treatment of telangiectasia and skin tags gives an excellent result with less trauma to the skin. The healing time for the skin is shorter than when using short-wave diathermy and pinprick scabs, where the needle has been inserted, are less likely to occur providing the balance of the two currents is correct.

A thorough consultation and patch test are essential before starting the main treatment.

The treatment of telangiectasia (red veins, broken capillaries)

Treatment steps

1 The area should be cleansed thoroughly before treatment to remove any traces of make-up, then wiped over with medi-wipes, weak hibitaine solution, tea tree solution or similar to ensure that the area is free from traces of cream, oil, germs and bacteria. It is not advisable to use surgical spirit, which is extremely drying to the skin.

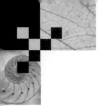

2 Surface anaesthetic can be applied to the treatment site when a client has a very low pain threshold. Emla cream should be applied at least 1 hour before treatment; alternatively, Amnitop can be applied at least 30 minutes before treatment. However, it should be remembered that Amnitop is a vasodilator, which may hinder the coagulation of the capillaries although smaller capillaries will become more visible and will therefore make insertion of the needle easier. The indifferent electrode should be covered with either damp cotton wool or a wet wipe and given to the client to hold. The use of the cotton wool not only encourages good conduction of the galvanic current, particularly when the skin is lacking in moisture, but also guards against a build up of hydrochloric acid on the hand and a subsequent galvanic burn.

3 The next step is to select the needle and open the packet in front of the client, unless the client has a phobia of needles.

A. Hair follicle

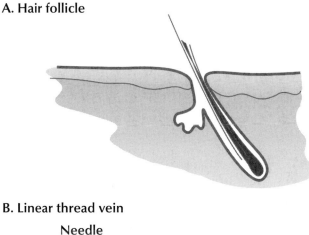

B. Linear thread vein

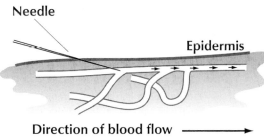

C. Spider naevi-central arteriole or Campbell de Morgan spot

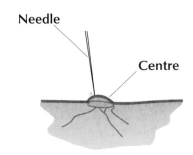

Figure 11.1
Angle of needle insertion in different applications

4   Establish the feeder capillary by gently stroking the vein along its length, watching very carefully to see the direction of blood flow in the capillaries. The aim of the treatment is to form a blood clot in the capillary to stop the flow of blood whilst at the same time coagulating the capillary walls.

5   Set the high frequency intensity to low and the galvanic (DC) to 0.2–0.3 milliamperes. Turn on the galvanic current only and insert the needle into the centre of the capillary. The use of galvanic current during insertion will gently dissolve the skin and allow easy penetration into the capillary.

6   After the needle has been inserted, apply a low intensity of high frequency current in conjunction with the galvanic current. The capillary will quickly turn white as coagulation takes place. Allow the combined currents to flow for 1–3 seconds or until capillary coagulation is no longer visible.

7   When coagulation is complete, turn off the high frequency current but allow the galvanic current to flow for a further 1–2 seconds without removing the needle. This has the action of producing sodium hydroxide in the blood clot, so dissolving sufficient coagulated matter to allow the needle to slide easily out of the skin without dislodging the clot. The skin should not stick to the needle when it is being withdrawn.

8   Do not treat too many capillaries in one area but allow sufficient healing space.

9   At the end of the treatment, dispose of the needle in a sharps box.

10   Apply aftercare and fully explain the home care procedure to the client. Follow this up with written instructions (see Chapter 9).

The treatment of spider naevi (spider telangiectasia)

A spider naevus has a central arteriole or capillary from which radiate small, fine capillaries, the appearance of which is reminiscent of a spider.

This treatment technique differs from the technique used for linear telangiectasia.

With the galvanic current on, gently insert the needle directly into the centre of the main arteriole or capillary (the central capillary is usually raised). Allow both galvanic and high frequency currents to flow until the centre is coagulated.

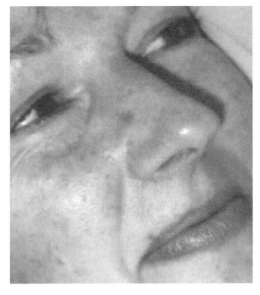

Coagulation of spider naevi often takes longer to achieve in comparison with thread/linear telangiectasia. Once coagulation has been achieved, turn off the high frequency and withdraw the needle whilst the galvanic current is still flowing.

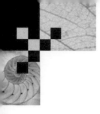

In many instances, it is not necessary to treat the fine radiating capillaries once the centre has been successfully coagulated. This is due to the fact that fine capillaries are often fed from the central capillary. Spider telangiectasia often need more than one treatment before they finally disappear.

A small scab may appear where the needle has been inserted into the spider telangiectasia. The client should be advised not to pick this off but to allow the scab to drop off naturally, which will usually occur within a few days.

The appearance of the skin after blend treatment

The skin's appearance after blend treatment will be similar to that of short-wave diathermy. However, there is less likelihood of small scabs appearing and the surface of the skin heals faster, returning to normal sooner. The application of cataphoresis after treatment will hasten the healing process. The erythema will subside in a shorter period of time and, in addition, the skin's natural pH balance will be restored. The action of the electrode has a soothing effect on both the skin and the client.

The application of cataphoresis after blend treatment

The application of cataphoresis (application of the positive pole) helps to reduce localised swelling and encourages vasoconstriction of the blood capillaries so reducing erythema at the treatment site. This procedure helps to bring about a localised reduction in skin temperature after treatment. Cataphoresis also helps to restore the skin's natural pH balance, thereby speeding up the healing process. This addition to the basic treatment is relaxing for the client leaving her or him with a sense of well-being.

Cataphoresis can be applied using a roller over an aloe-based gel or a pad of cotton wool soaked with witch hazel. The electrode is then gently rolled over the treatment site for approximately 4–5 minutes at a DC setting of 0.5–1.00 milliamperes. Care must be taken to avoid applying too much pressure during the process otherwise the roller could open the coagulated areas.

The removal of skin tags with blend

Skin tags can be removed with less trauma to the skin by using the blend technique.

Treatment steps

1 Gently lift the skin tag away from the skin with sterile tweezers.
2 Using galvanic current only, insert the needle into the neck of the skin tag, between the skin surface and body of the skin tag.
3 Apply both high frequency and galvanic currents. Allow the currents to flow until the tag begins to dissolve.

4 When sufficient current has been applied, the tag can be lifted away from the skin.

5 The area will appear slightly red with a little swelling. This will settle down within 24 hours. The skin will heal within the next 2 weeks.

The removal of Campbell de Morgan spots (cherry angioma)

These are usually found on the chest, back and sometimes the arms. They are red, raised, and round in appearance. These angiomas consist of a number of small closely grouped capillaries, which protrude from the dermis into the epidermis.

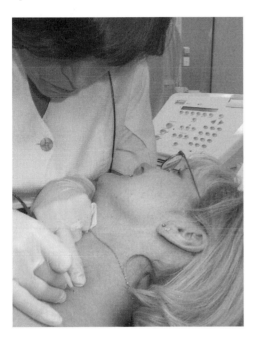 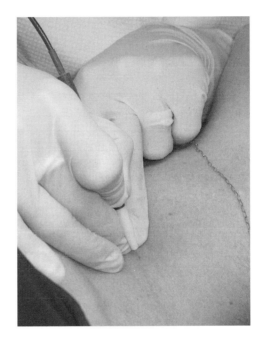

Treatment steps

1 Select a size 3 or 4 telangiectasia needle, depending on the size of the angioma.

2 With the galvanic current flowing, gently insert the needle into the angioma.

3 Apply the galvanic and high frequency currents simultaneously until coagulation starts to take place.

4 Depending on the size of the angioma, it may be necessary to carry out several insertions to achieve full coagulation.

5 The colour of the angioma changes to dark red or black as the blood is coagulated. A crust will form over the treatment site. This will fall off during the following week.

6 Depending on the size of the angioma, it may be necessary to carry out several treatments to achieve the desired result.

7 Apply aftercare.

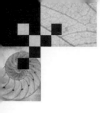

The causes of scarring when using blend

When too much galvanic current is used during treatment, there will be a build up of sodium hydroxide (lye) within the skin. Sodium hydroxide is extremely caustic and will effectively dissolve tissue. If too much is produced, not only will the capillary be destroyed but also the surrounding tissue, which will result in unsightly pit marks (skin necrosis), which may well be permanent. Weeping of lymph will occur at the treatment site and in time crusts will form. If these crusts are picked off by the client, deep pit marks will be left. Again, these could be permanent. Too much galvanic current will result in sore, swollen skin that is painful to the touch. This may take several weeks to subside.

When too much high frequency is used, tenting of the skin around the needle can occur. This will lead to scabbing and skin necrosis. White marks at the point of insertion may appear. Too much heat applied near the surface will result in pigmentation marks.

Summary

The combined application of galvanic and high frequency currents can be used for the treatment of telangiectasia and spider telangiectasia, Campbell de Morgan spots, as well as the removal of skin tags. The healing time for the skin is shorter than when using short-wave diathermy and pinprick scabs where the needle has been inserted are less likely to occur, providing the balance of the two currents is correct.

The galvanic current is used to gently dissolve the skin when the needle is inserted; high frequency coagulates the blood to form a clot, and when the needle is withdrawn from the clot a small amount of galvanic current is used to slightly dissolve the clot around the needle. This prevents the clot from being dislodged when the needle is removed.

Review questions

1 List the benefits of applying cataphoreses at the end of the removal of telangiectasia with blend.

2 Describe how the skin should appear after blend treatment.

3 List the benefits of blend for the removal of telangiectasia and skin tags.

4 List the causes of scarring as a result of blend application to the skin.

5 State the DC intensity that should be used for the treatment of telangiectasia.

6 Explain the disadvantages of using too much high frequency current when using blend technique.

7 What is the advantage of using a needle that has been designed specifically for the treatment of telangiectasia?

8 Why is the needle withdrawn from the skin with the galvanic current still flowing?

9 How does the treatment of a spider telangiectasia differ from the treatment of linear telangiectasia?

Chapter 12

Sclerotherapy

Key points

1 Sclerotherapy has been shown to be the most effective method of removing spider thread veins from the legs.

2 Sclerotherapy can be used in combination with laser or intense pulsed light.

3 A comprehensive consultation is essential prior to treatment, and a signed consent form must be obtained from the client.

4 The procedure involves the injection of a small amount of **sclerosing fluid** into the vein.

5 Clients should be advised that the full benefits of a sclerotherapy procedure may not be seen for 6–8 weeks.

Thread veins on the legs are extremely common and cause embarrassment and distress for many women. An experienced electrolysist using short-wave diathermy or blend can successfully treat facial telangiectasia. However, this method of treatment has been found to be ineffective on the leg area. For this area sclerotherapy is the preferred method, usually reducing thread veins by 60–80 per cent over 2–4 treatments. There are considerable variations in the results depending on such factors as the size of the thread veins, the length of time the thread veins have been present, and the skill of the operator. Permanent improvements by sclerotherapy cannot be guaranteed unless the cause is removed. However, clients are generally pleased with the results.

Women attending for sclerotherapy are often looking for the complete elimination of all unsightly thread veins, not only permanently but also in time for next week's holiday. Alas, perfection is not possible and it is important to set expectations at realistic levels. Sadly, clients do not always want to hear this and the point needs to be reinforced in order to avoid disappointment. The importance of a full consultation including detailed information on the limitations, complications and results that are likely to arise from the treatment cannot be stressed too strongly. Without the relevant information, the risk of having an unhappy client rises dramatically as does the likelihood of generating work for your solicitor.

Spider thread veins on the legs often occur in association with varicose veins. It is frequently an inherited problem that is aggravated by pregnancy, occupations involving prolonged periods of standing (e.g. hairdressing) or sitting, obesity and the taking of hormones such as Hormone Replacement Therapy (HRT).

The consultation

A comprehensive consultation is essential prior to treatment, and a signed consent form must be obtained from the client. It is always advisable to take photographs prior to treatment for two reasons.

1 Due to the treatment being spread over a number of sessions, it is often difficult for the client to remember the extent of the problem before treatment.

2 Photographs provide a record of progress and show the exact site of the problem. There are times when a client is convinced that the veins have reappeared and that treatment has not been successful, when, in reality, new veins have appeared in close proximity to those previously treated.

The sclerotherapy procedure should be explained in detail at this stage. Clients will want to know what the treatment will feel like and whether it is painful. How many treatments will be needed? The latter is a commonly asked question that is difficult to answer. There is a considerable variation in response between one individual and another, therefore, as with epilation treatment, it is advisable to avoid giving an exact number of treatments required. Explain the role of the sclerosing solution and provide information on the side effects that can occur Clients should also be made aware of the appearance of the area immediately after treatment and the subsequent appearance/changes that will take place during the course of the following few weeks.

The aftercare procedure should also be explained during the consultation and written instructions given to the client; the receipt of which should be signed for by the client at the time of treatment.

Contra-indications

During the consultation, it is necessary to check for contra-indications, which include:

◆ varicose veins – best dealt with before treating thread veins as the increased pressure within the venous system is likely to give an unsuccessful outcome. If the client has had surgery for varicose veins, treatment should be delayed for 3 months

◆ a medical history of clotting disorders including venous thrombosis

◆ haemophilia

◆ use of anticoagulant drugs, e.g. warfarin

◆ caution must be observed in patients on NSIADs for arthritis and low dose aspirin, both of which cause bleeding tendencies

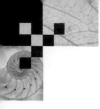

◆ poorly controlled diabetes

◆ significant heart disease

◆ use of oral steroid medication (Prednisolone)

◆ severe obesity

◆ a history of leg ulceration

◆ pregnancy – it is important to ask about the client's last menstrual period to avoid treatment during pregnancy.

Often the decision to treat or not rests on weighing up a number of factors and the responsibility for such decisions lies with the authorising doctor. The above list is not intended to give a comprehensive breakdown of contra-indications but provides more of a general overview.

Sclerotherapy procedure

Sclerotherapy is the procedure whereby a very small amount of sclerosing chemical solution is injected into the vein. Blanching will occur as the solution flows into the vein. Practising sclerotherapists refer to this as the 'flush' – a momentary and very satisfying sight for the therapist as the thread veins are seen to disappear when the solution enters the vein.

The sclerosing fluid is a chemical irritant, which has the effect of irritating the vein wall, causing it to become inflamed and swollen, then thrombosed, leading to the death of the vein. The blood stops flowing through the vein, and over a period of up to 8 weeks the remains of the vein will become absorbed by the body's immune system once it recognises that the vein has been damaged. There are a number of sclerosing solutions available for injection (on prescription only) with minor differences, therefore the preference is entirely with the prescribing physician.

Treatment by sclerotherapy should be confined to the legs although many doctors now perform sclerotherapy on the face. It would be wise to keep in mind the case published by the Medical Defence Union of a doctor who was successfully sued because of necrosis and subsequent scarring at the injection site on a client's face. Treatment by short-wave diathermy or blend on the face has proved to be very effective when performed by a skilled and *experienced* electrolysist.

Small thread veins are often technically difficult to inject by virtue of their small diameter and it may well be only the more skilled and experienced operators who are successful with these veins. On the other hand, heavy thread veins, which are wide-bored and have been present for some time, may well require modification of the injection technique with more emphasis on holding the solution in the vein just after the vein has been flushed and the application of compression after the treatment in the form of an elasticated bandage. Many of the clients presenting for treatment will have small thread veins and it is for precisely this reason that *experienced, skilled practising* electrolysists are so successful. They possess the necessary skills, with a magnifying lens and light, combined with the necessary hand and eye co-ordination, to perform accurate injections.

The appearance of skin after sclerotherapy treatment

During treatment the solution will cause blanching along the vein. Within a few minutes of treatment, the area around the veins will be pink or red and become swollen, similar to a nettle sting. Bruising may occur at the site but will be short lived. The initial reaction settles within 24–48 hours. The area may be slightly itchy. The vein usually gets darker in colour and the thicker the vein, the darker it will appear after treatment. At the site of the injection, where the needle punctures the vein, a small amount of blood may leak under the skin and cause a small area of pigmentation. This usually fades, but in some cases can take many months to do so. As the vein disappears, a faint brown line may be left rather like a tea stain which will also eventually fade.

Side effects of sclerotherapy

◆ The formation of new minute blood vessels called 'telangiectactic matting' can occur. These will respond better when treated by laser, intense pulsed light, short-wave diathermy or blend.

◆ Ulceration at the site of the injection is due to extravasation of fluid outside the vessel. This requires prompt medical treatment as it can produce permanent scarring.

◆ Mild thrombophlebitis can occur for a few days and needs treatment with compression bandages.

◆ Ankle oedema is particularly likely in those clients who have a past history of fluid retention.

◆ The most serious potential problem is an allergic reaction to the chemical irritant. This can take the form of a skin rash or more seriously anaphylactic shock (**anaphylaxis**).

Anaphylactic shock (anaphylaxis)

Many electrolysists are familiar with the term 'anaphylactic shock' but are not fully conversant with its meaning. Anaphylactic shock is a rare, potentially life-threatening occurrence of which all in the beauty therapy/electrology fields should be aware. The media have alerted the general public to the problem by highlighting the increasing incidence of anaphylactic shock, particularly in children allergic to nut products.

Therapists working in their clinics/salons could encounter anaphylaxis in almost any aspect of the treatments they are providing; even a simple facial could trigger a reaction in someone who is sensitive to the materials used. However, with invasive procedures, such as sclerotherapy or collagen replacement therapy,

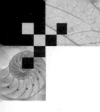

the risk of rapid onset of anaphylactic shock is greater. Although there are no recorded cases of severe reaction to sclerotherapy, the large increase in the number of these procedures being performed in salons raises the statistical chance of it occurring.

Anaphylactic shock is a severe allergic reaction that occurs rapidly when the immune system is exposed to a specific substance to which it has been previously sensitised. The allergy-causing substance enters the bloodstream and triggers the release of chemicals throughout the body that are trying to protect it from foreign substances. It is the release of these chemicals that leads to the symptoms of anaphylactic shock.

Symptoms

The initial symptoms may occur within minutes of exposure depending on the method of administration of the substance.

Symptoms include:

- generalised itching of the skin and a raised rash (hives)
- flushing and swelling of the lips, throat, hands, tongue and feet
- wheezing, shortness of breath, coughing and hoarseness
- headache, nausea, vomiting and abdominal cramps
- loss of consciousness.

If the above symptoms develop, treatment must be discontinued immediately and the following plan adopted.

1 Adrenalin should be administered if available (only by a qualified practitioner legally permitted to carry out this procedure).
2 If unconscious, place the client in the recovery position.
3 Summon help by dialing 999.
4 Do not leave the client unattended at any time.

The presence of adrenalin in salons will depend on the type of therapies being undertaken. Those salons/clinic performing invasive procedures such as sclerotherapy should have access to the Epipen system. This is a simple injection device designed for those suffering from anaphylactic shock, which can be used speedily and efficiently.

Reducing the risks of anaphylactic shock

Although such a severe allergic reaction is rare, to minimise the risk, it is of vital importance to select clients carefully prior to treatment. A clear and detailed medical history, including specific enquiries into any allergic or anaphylactic reactions, must be taken and those clients found to be sensitive excluded from sclerotherapy treatment.

Legal requirements

Sclerotherapy is a medical procedure, which may be delegated by a doctor to another professional. It is important for electrolysists to remember that the doctor retains an overall responsibility for the management of the client; that an electrolysist must *never* treat a client without first discussing the client's medical history with the supervising doctor and gaining the appropriate authorisation to proceed. Electrolysists who attempt sclerotherapy without first getting the approval of a supervising doctor, place themselves outside the law and render their professional indemnity insurance null and void.

Clinics practising the removal of telangiectasia on the face will find that they receive numerous enquiries concerning the removal of thread veins on the legs. Some electrolysists are tempted to think of this as a good source of income and rush to find the first available training course. There are a number of courses available but careful research into the training establishments and their reputations should be undertaken prior to making a commitment.

Sclerotherapy treatment carries a high degree of responsibility. Not every electrolysist has the necessary skill or patience to undertake this field of work. The repercussions arising from poor quality treatment can be horrendous, not to mention extremely lucrative for the solicitors involved should legal action be taken against the electrolysist.

Sclerotherapy for thread veins: client information

When a client attends the clinic for the initial consultation it is advisable to give her or him a 'client information sheet' that she or he can read at home. The sheet should include brief information on the treatment, procedure, and answers to questions most commonly asked by clients.

The following has been reprinted by kind permission of Dr Mervyn Patterson of Woodford Medical Services.

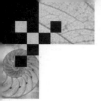

Sclerotherapy for thread veins

Client Information

1 Sclerotherapy involves the use of a tiny needle to flush a small amount of medication into the thread veins to cause them to dissolve away.

2 It is not possible to get rid of every thread vein but we will try to decrease the venous appearance of your legs with gradual lightening of the thread veins with each session.

3 A very slight pricking sensation may be felt as the injections are being performed.

4 After the first day of treatment, the skin around the vein is a little pink and blotchy. Occasionally, people with more sensitive skin see more pinkness or reaction around the veins. Usually a bruise is noticeable at the treated site. This usually disappears after a few weeks but in some cases may take months to fade.

5 A length of tubigrip will be used to cover the treated areas after injection. This should be left on for 24 hours.

6 Creams, oils, lotions, tanning or perfumed products should not be used on the area on the day or during the next 48 hours.

7 Hot baths or showers should be avoided, as should the use of additional bath products for 48 hours.

8 Avoid prolonged sitting, standing, pounding types of exercise, squatting and heavy weight lifting after the treatment. You are encouraged to walk after the treatment.

9 Avoid alcohol and aspirins for 24 hours before and after treatment.

10 Possible complications of sclerotherapy include:

   ◆ pigmentation – a result of staining caused by small amounts of blood just under the skin surface. These normally fade very quickly but in some cases may take some months to disappear

   ◆ scarring/staining – some feint brown marks may be left by the vein walls as they are dissolving. These gradually fade but this may take several months

   ◆ telangiectatic matting – very fine, small, blushed capillaries left as larger thread veins regress

   ◆ skin necrosis – a shallow ulcer can occur at the site of the injection. This is very unusual and always heals

   ◆ allergic reactions – are very unlikely and have not been reported with the solution your therapist uses.

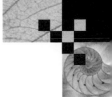

Summary

Sclerotherapy is the preferred method for treating spider thread veins on the legs. A 60–80 per cent improvement in the appearance of these veins is possible with between 2–4 treatment sessions depending upon the severity of the condition.

Clients should receive a full consultation prior to treatment. This should cover medical background, possible causes of the thread veins, an explanation of the treatment procedure, the skin's appearance immediately after treatment, and the changes that will occur in the following 8 weeks. Side effects and contra-indications should also be discussed. Before and after photographs will help the client to remember how the veins looked before treatment; it is surprising how soon they forget, and in many instances are convinced that there has not been any improvement.

Sclerotherapy is a medical procedure that is carried out by doctors, nurses and some electrolysists. The doctor retains overall responsibility for the client.

The procedure involves the injection of a small amount of sclerosing fluid into the vein. Initially, a flushing of the vein can be seen as the solution is introduced. The function of the solution is to irritate the walls of the vein, which become inflamed and thrombosed, causing the death of the vein. Blood can no longer flow through the vein and when the vein dies it is absorbed by the body's immune system.

There are a few side effects associated with sclerotherapy. These are brown pigmentation marks where the solution has leaked at the site of the injections, capillary matting, ulceration where the needle has been inserted into the vein, mild thrombophlebitis and anaphylactic shock.

Anaphylactic shock (anaphylaxis) is a severe allergic reaction that occurs rapidly when the immune system is exposed to a specific substance to which it has been previously sensitised. The allergy-causing substance enters the bloodstream and triggers the release of chemicals throughout the body that are trying to protect it from foreign substances. Adrenalin should be administered immediately. A person who is prone to anaphylactic shock will normally carry an Epipen with them at all times.

Sclerotherapy can be used in conjunction with other treatments such as laser, intense pulsed light and electrolysis for very fine capillaries.

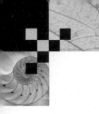

Review questions

1   Define 'sclerotherapy'.

2   Why is sclerotherapy more effective for treating superficial leg veins than the blend or short-wave diathermy techniques?

3   Why is it not advisable to use sclerotherapy for facial telangiectasia?

4   What is meant by the term 'capillary matting'?

5   List five side effects of sclerotherapy.

6   List six contra-indications to sclerotherapy.

7   Explain the home care instructions that should be given to clients who have received sclerotherapy.

8   What is anaphylatic shock?

9   Describe the treatment for anaphylactic shock.

Intense pulsed light

Key points

1 Intense pulsed light (IPL) is a non-invasive method of treating vascular conditions from simple telangiectasia and spider naevi to the more complex port wine stains.

2 Intense pulsed light effectively removes vascular lesions by selective photothermolysis.

3 The health and condition of the skin has an influence on the treatment result.

4 Blood vessels will appear darker immediately after treatment.

5 Clients must be questioned with regard to any change of medication, contra-indications and exposure to sunlight at the beginning of every treatment.

6 Treatment should not be given when a client has had exposure to sunlight without the use of a high factor sun barrier, regardless of how short the sunlight exposure was, as *the skin will burn or blister, even after the shortest exposure.*

In comparison to other techniques of electrical epilation, lasers and intense pulsed light (IPL) systems are relatively new treatments for pigmentation disorders, vascular disturbances and the removal of benign skin lesions. IPL has been used since the 1990s, and lasers since the 1960s. The therapist should understand the difference between the two methods, their application and home care advice, but should also be able to give a clear description of the skin's appearance whilst healing is taking place. The therapist should have knowledge of the contra-indications and be aware of possible side effects. It is not feasible to cover the subject in depth in this text. The aim is to give a general overview so that the therapist can discuss the subject with clients in an informed manner.

Laser light is known as a **coherent**, **monochromatic**, **collimated** light, which is non-divergent, and the beam can be maintained over long distances. To put it more simply, the light emitted from a laser is very nearly parallel (collimated); the waves travel in phase with one another in an ordered manner. Intense pulsed light (IPL) is a white light source that is often confused with laser, particularly by prospective clients.

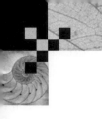

Intense pulsed light	Laser
Polychromatic light	Monochromatic light
Variable wavelengths	Fixed wavelength
Non-coherent	Coherent
Divergent	Non-divergent
Non-collimated	Collimated

Table 13.1 Comparison between IPL and laser light

Intense pulsed light is a non-invasive, non-collimated, non-coherent light source of variable ***wavelengths***. The treatment works by selective photothermolysis, which can be defined as follows:

Selective   – targets specific ***chromophores***, e.g. melanin or haemaglobin

Photo   – light

Thermolysis – destruction by heat.

IPL is a versatile treatment that is used for the treatment of benign vascular disorders, pigmentation marks and long-term hair removal. The flexibility of ***pulse duration***, application of single or multiple pulses, ***fluence*** (energy) and pulse delay allow the operator to adjust or set treatment parameters according to the needs of the individual. Conditions that may be treated effectively with intense pulsed light include:

- facial telangiectasia
- haemangiomas
- spider naevi
- capillary matting
- fine thread veins on the legs
- cafe au lait spots
- port wine stains.

Contra-indications

The literal meaning of the term 'contra-indication' is *an indication against treatment*. There are a number of contra-indications to intense pulsed light treatment. They include:

- recent exposure to sunlight – active melanin cells within the skin
- the use of sunbeds 4–6 weeks prior to IPL treatment

◆ diabetes – bruises easily, slow to heal if problems should occur

◆ active epilepsy – flashes of light may bring on an attack

◆ photosensitive skin

◆ photosensitive medication, including herbal remedies such as St John's Wort

◆ pregnancy

◆ asthma – a recent attack where an excess of steroids and inotropes are given may still be in the body

◆ moles – best avoided because it is difficult to determine whether they are benign, pre-malignant or malignant

◆ haemophilia – faulty clotting mechanism

◆ kidney infections (short term just while infection is present) – fluid retention may be present

◆ herpes simplex that arises as a result of exposure to sunlight (treatment site only)

◆ dysmorphobia.

Skin assessment before treatment

The condition of the skin influences the treatment result. It is essential that the client is asked specific questions before every treatment.

1 Has there been any change in health? If the answer is 'yes', more detailed questions must be asked concerning the changes before deciding whether treatment should be postponed to a later date.

2 Has the client been prescribed medication; if so, is the medication photosensitive?

3 Has the client been exposed to ultraviolet light without using a sun protection product of at least factor 30, even for 5 minutes? Often clients do not consider spending time in the garden, shopping or driving in the car when the sun is shining as exposure to sunlight!

4 Is the skin very dry? This will affect the absorption of light into the skin.

5 Is there a hint of tan on the skin?

6 Has the client used artificial tanning products within the previous 10 days?

Treatment should not be given if the client gives a positive answer to any of the above. The application of intense pulsed light, when any of the above exists, could result in adverse reactions such as hypo- or hyper-pigmentation, blistering, superficial burns and scabbing. Hyper-pigmentation (increased) will gradually fade over a period of time but it could take several months, whereas hypo-pigmentation (loss) may well be permanent.

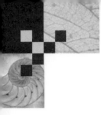

Treatment procedure

Treatment steps

1 After the relevant questions have been asked and the area cleansed, the operator chooses the correct fluence (energy), the number of pulses per shot, the pulse duration and pulsed delay.

2 Cold, non-pigmented gel is applied to the treatment site. The purpose of this gel is to protect the epidermis from the heat of the IPL whilst at the same time allowing the passage of light into the dermis.

3 The treatment head is held so that the filter rests on the surface of the gel but does not make direct contact with the skin. The light is delivered to the treatment site either in single or multiple pulses. When the light is delivered to the skin, the client will feel a slight stinging sensation similar to a splash of hot fat from a frying pan or the twang of a rubber band. The sensation lasts for a fraction of a second.

4 The gel, which will now be warm, is then removed from the skin.

5 Cool packs may be applied to the area if required.

6 Aftercare in the form of aloe vera gel, witch hazel gel or a similar preparation is applied to the area immediately after treatment.

7 The client's skin reaction should be noted and entered into the client's record card together with the treatment parameters that have been used.

8 Detailed verbal and written home care instructions should then be given to the client.

The appearance of the skin immediately after treatment

Immediately after treatment there will be erythema and mild oedema. The skin may also feel warm for a short period of time. The sensation is one that can be compared to sun exposure without a suitable sunscreen.

Blood vessels: immediately after treatment the vessel will appear darker. Erythema and oedema will be present around the vessel. Vasoconstriction will occur and the vessel will either disappear or become darker for a short period of time.

Pigmented lesions: initially, there is a greying or darkening of the lesion and there will also be oedema around the lesion.

Process of clearance

Blood: phagocytes eliminate clots and wall debris.

Melanin particles: from pigmented lesions or hair bulbs and debris are also phagocytised.

The time taken for the lesions to clear after treatment will vary from one person to another. However, it does not happen overnight, or immediately after treatment. The absorption of vascular and pigmented debris takes time and is dependant on the size of the lesion or vessel, the concentration of pigment, and the physiological condition of the skin. Clients should be advised that it could take up to 2 months for the full benefits of the treatment to be seen.

Adverse skin reactions

There are a number of reasons why adverse skin reactions can occur. However, skin reactions are rare when all precautions are taken prior to treatment and the correct procedure and parameters applied.

Side effects include:

- marking, or stripes – which match the footprint of the filter
- blisters
- scabbing and crusting – particularly in darker skins
- hyper- or hypo-pigmentation
- scars.

All the above will be temporary, with the exception of loss of pigmentation. The pigmentation may eventually return; however, it will be a very slow process, taking up to 18 months or more.

Post-treatment/home care

The area must be kept cool but advise against the application of ice directly onto the skin. A soothing cream such as aloe vera should be applied regularly. Sometimes the client may feel a burning sensation in which case an after burns cream should be applied. Steroid or antibiotic creams can be prescribed if the skin is lacerated or blistered.

Clients should be advised to avoid aerobic exercise and hot baths for at least 48 hours. Steam and heat treatments should be avoided until the skin has healed completely and it is preferable that make-up is not used for up to 7 days if possible. Make-up should not be applied over blistered skin or open wounds. Exposure to sunlight without a complete sunblock must be avoided for a minimum of 6 weeks.

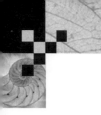

Summary

IPL is a relatively new technology that is proving to be very effective in the treatment of pigment lesions and vascular disturbances such as telangiectasia, spider naevi and port wine stains. IPL is a white light source from the visible light spectrum.

The treatment works by selective photothermolysis, targeting the melanin pigment in the skin and haemoglobin in the blood. When applied correctly, side effects are rare. However, burns, hypo-pigmentation and hyper-pigmentation can occur. The lesions do not disappear immediately after treatment and it can take up to 2 months for the results to be seen.

The skin may be warm immediately after treatment and erythema and oedema may be present. Blood vessels may disappear immediately or may appear darker in colour, gradually fading within 2 months.

There are several contra-indications which must be checked out thoroughly before treatment is given to avoid adverse skin reaction and a disappointed client.

Review questions

1   Compare laser light with intense pulsed light.

2   Define the term 'intense pulsed light'.

3   What is meant by the term 'selective photothermolysis'?

4   List five conditions that can be treated with intense pulsed light.

5   List the contra-indications to intense pulsed light.

6   State the questions that a client should be asked by the electrolysist before every treatment.

7   Describe the treatment procedure using intense pulsed light.

8   Give the home care routine that the client should follow after treatment.

9   Describe the appearance of: a) blood vessels and b) pigmentation marks after treatment.

10   List four possible adverse skin reactions to intense pulsed light.

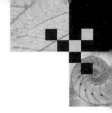

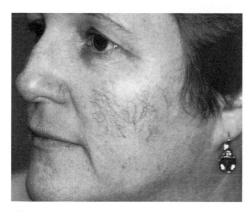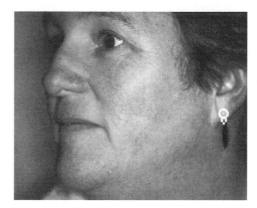

Figure 13.1 Female with telangiectasia before and after three IPL treatments

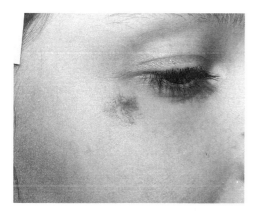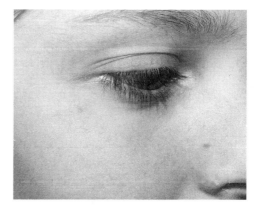

Figure 13.2 Female with broken veins before and after four IPL treatments

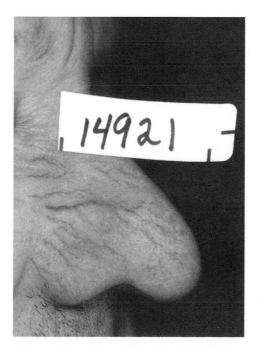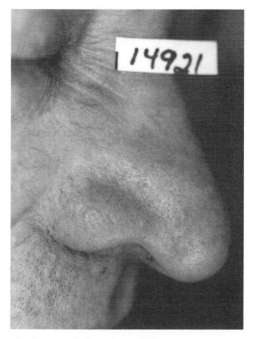

Figure 13.3 Male with telangiectasia (on nose) before and after three IPL treatments

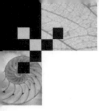

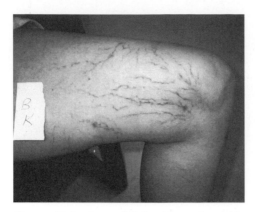 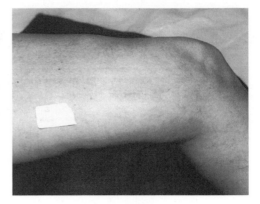

Figure 13.4   Superficial spider veins (skin type IV) before and after one IPL treatment

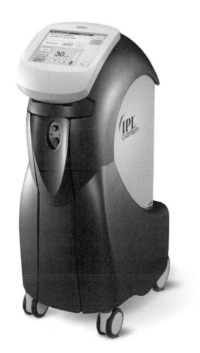 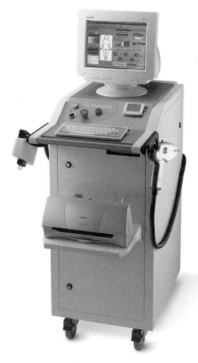

Figure 13.5   Quantum IPL machine   **Figure 13.6**   Lumenis Vasculight, right view

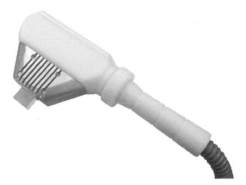 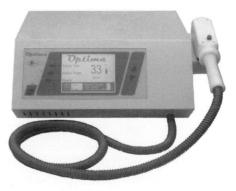

Figure 13.7   CTI Optima   **Figure 13.8**   CTI Optima

Laser treatments for benign vascular lesions

Chapter 14

Key points

1 Clients' expectations of treatment results are often unrealistic.

2 Laser is an anacronym for Light Amplification for the Stimulated Emission of Radiation.

3 Laser treatment can be combined with sclerotherapy and intense pulsed light when treating leg veins.

4 The target chromaphore is haemoglobin when treating vascular lesions and abnormalities.

5 The aim of treatment is to coagulate the blood in the veins by selective photothermolysis.

6 The client should receive a full consultation prior to laser treatment.

Laser treatment for vascular disorders

Lasers caught the imagination of the general public in the late 1990s for many treatments such as hair removal, laser resurfacing for the removal of wrinkles, fine lines, superficial acne scars or the removal of facial thread veins, leg veins and other vascular malformations such as haemangiomas and port wine stains. Clients' expectations of the treatment results are often unrealistic. To avoid disappointment, it is essential that all clients receive a thorough consultation and explanation of the procedure and possible results prior to treatment.

Clients expect their electrolysist to be fully conversant with the range of treatments available for telangiectasia and vascular malformations whether it is electrical epilation (with either short-wave diathermy or blend), laser, intense pulsed light or sclerotherapy.

To give the electrolysist an insight into how lasers can be used to treat vascular conditions such as telangiectasia, spider naevi, and superficial leg veins this chapter will give an overview of:

◆ basic terminology associated with lasers

◆ lasers in the use of vascular disorders and how they work

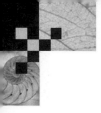

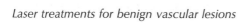

- ◆ the interaction of laser light on skin tissue
- ◆ laser action on blood vessels
- ◆ the skin's reaction and appearance after treatment
- ◆ the healing procedure
- ◆ home care recommendations
- ◆ contra-indications.

Laser is an acronym for:

L – light

A – amplification of

S – stimulated

E – emission of

R – radiation.

Albert Einstein predicted the possibility of generating laser light as early as 1917, but it was not until the late 1950s and early 60s that his forecast became a reality.

Laser light can be described as the monochromatic, collimated, coherent, non-ionising radiation of a fixed wavelength.

There are a number of definitions associated with lasers that the operator should be familiar with.

Chromaphore: is the term given to the light-absorbing target, e.g. melanin in hair removal and haemoglobin in the blood.

Pulse duration: refers to the length of time the laser light is on the tissue.

Fluence: is the amount of energy delivered to a unit area in a single pulse.

Monochromatic: refers to the ability of laser energy to emit light in a single wavelength of a specific colour, e.g. pulsed dye laser produces a yellow light, whereas the KTP laser produces a green light.

Collimated: wavelengths are emitted in parallel to one another without divergence as the beam travels through space.

Coherence: is defined as light waves that are spatially and temporally in phase with one another. The properties of coherence and collimation allow the laser energy to be focused accurately in a very small beam of light, e.g. energy fluence.

Energy fluence: is the amount of energy delivered to a unit area in a single pulse and is measured in joules or watts per cm².

Lasers used for therapeutic purposes work within the visible light spectrum ranging from ultraviolet to near infrared.

How lasers work when treating blood vessels

The aim of the treatment, as with intense pulsed light, is to coagulate the blood vessels by selective photothermolysis. Treatment by laser therapy is successful because the wavelength of the laser used targets the red haemoglobin in the blood. The blood takes up the heat from the laser light and is coagulated (selective photothermolysis).

The interaction of laser light on skin tissue and blood vessels

Laser light of a fixed wavelength, e.g. 532 nm, emits a green light that is absorbed by the target chromaphore, in this instance, haemoglobin. When the energy is absorbed by the chromophore (it is known that haemoglobin absorbs green light), the temperature within the tissue is raised to a temperature of 60–70°C. The lining of the blood vessels will be thermally damaged and shrink. At the same time, blood will be coagulated resulting in a clot or thrombus. In this way the flow of blood is interrupted.

The choice of laser depends on the type of vascular condition being treated. There are a number of lasers available.

The argon laser: works on wavelengths of 480 nm emitting a blue light, or 514 nm emitting a green light.

The pulsed dye laser: works at a wavelength of 585 nm producing a yellow light and is mainly used by the medical profession for the removal of port wine stains, strawberry naevi and birthmarks.

The NdYag pulsed Q switched laser: works at a wavelength of 1064 nm and produces near infrared light. This laser is effective on deeper blue leg veins (not varicose veins) and blue spider thread veins in the legs.

The KTP double frequency NdYag: works at a wavelength of 532 nm, producing a green light. This is the most popular laser for the treatment of facial telangiectasia, spider naevi, diffused flushing of the cheeks and nose, and poikiloderma.

Treatment procedure

A facial laser treatment can include both cheeks, nose and chin and would normally take no longer than 30–45 minutes. The treatment of facial veins is relatively pain free. However, clients who are reluctant to have treatment without an anaesthetic can be prescribed a topical cream, such as Emla, to apply to the skin 1 hour before treatment. The sensation of a laser treatment can be described as a tingling or prickly sensation of short duration.

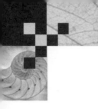

1 The skin is cooled with ice packs or cold compresses for a short time before treatment.

2 The settings are chosen and the treatment applied.

3 The treated area is cooled immediately afterwards with cold packs.

The skin's reaction to laser treatment and appearance afterwards

Following treatment, facial skin will feel a little hot and tender (similar to the feeling of slight sunburn) with slight swelling. With the correct aftercare, as recommended by the clinic, these symptoms will subside within 3–6 days. There may be some crusting, although this is rare, and it is important that this is allowed to fall off naturally. Under *no* circumstances should crusts be picked off otherwise scarring may occur.

The healing procedure time span

Facial veins

The healing time after the treatment of facial veins varies from one person to another. Initially, the skin will be warm to the touch and feel tender with some swelling. This may last for several days. Immediately after treatment the veins may appear to look worse than they did before treatment. During the following 7–10 days, the swelling will subside and the erythema will gradually fade. This process can take between 3–4 weeks to fade completely.

In very rare instances blistering can occur. Clients should always be warned about this possibility before commencing treatment. Any blistering that occurs usually heals within 7–10 days. However, clients should be told that they must not interfere with the skin and that they must follow the clinic's aftercare instructions. Clients should be invited to attend the clinic for a post-treatment consultation with the doctor or therapist 5–10 days after treatment.

Treatment sessions should be spaced at least 4–6 weeks apart. The frequency depends on the severity of the problem, the healing capacity of the skin and skin sensitivity.

Leg veins

When laser is applied to the vein, it is noticeable that the vein disappears. Within a short period of time, the vein appears slightly swollen with erythema in the immediate area.

During the next 7–14 days, the vein becomes darker in colour, then gradually starts to fade. This procedure may take as long as 6 weeks for some clients. The time span varies from one client to another, it is therefore advisable to make clients aware of the worst-case scenario.

Combined treatments

Leg veins

Laser, sclerotherapy and intense pulsed light for the treatment of leg veins can all be used as treatments in their own right. In many instances, the client will benefit from a combination of two or more.

Deeper veins can be treated with NdYag or KTP lasers whilst the smaller leg thread veins will respond well to sclerotherapy.

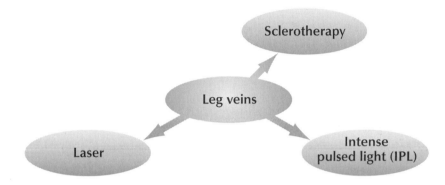

Figure 14.1

Sclerotherapy can sometimes leave an area of capillary matting or brown staining where the sclerosing solution has leaked from the vein. The application of intense pulsed light will help to resolve these problems.

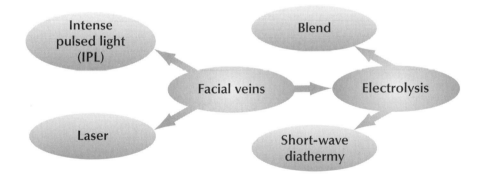

Figure 14.2

Facial veins

Facial capillaries respond well to treatment by electrolysis, using either blend or short-wave diathermy. Where an area of flushing is present and it is difficult to see the individual capillaries, intense pulsed light would be beneficial. Deeper capillaries and deep spider naevi that are difficult to treat with epilation will often respond well to laser treatment.

Home care

Correct home care plays an important role in the healing process. This must be fully explained to the client both before and after treatment. It is rare for clients to absorb all the verbal information that has been given to them, therefore written home care instructions should be issued to the client.

Facial veins

◆ Further cooling to the skin at home may be necessary. Cool packs wrapped in a clean cloth or a damp face cloth can be used.

◆ An aftercare soothing gel, such as aloe vera, should be given to clients to apply at home. This gel can be kept in the fridge in between applications.

◆ Clients should be advised that in some instances blistering or crusting may occur. These must not be interfered with but left to heal naturally. Picking at crusts could cause infection and/or subsequent scarring.

◆ The use of facial cleansers or cosmetics should be avoided for 48 hours following treatment or longer if the skin feels sensitive.

◆ Sun protection of at least factor 30 must be used at all times when the treated area is exposed to sunlight however minimal.

◆ Swimming and sports activities should be avoided until the skin has settled down. Heat, perspiration and stimulating facial circulation can cause irritation to the tissues and prolong the healing process.

◆ Clients should receive a follow-up telephone call to make sure that the treated area is settling satisfactorily.

◆ The client should return to the clinic after 4 weeks for a check-up and if necessary a further treatment session should be arranged.

◆ Clients should be invited to telephone the clinic if they are concerned or need clarification about their treatment or require further home care advice.

Leg veins

◆ Vigorous exercise should be avoided for 4–5 days.

◆ Swimming, saunas, heat treatments and the use of jacuzzis should be avoided for 48 hours.

◆ Body scrubs, friction and loofers should not be applied to the treatment site.

◆ Exposure to sunlight without total sunblock should be avoided to reduce the risk of pigmentation marks occurring.

◆ Self-tanning products and perfumed body lotions should not be applied for 48 hours.

◆ In the rare event of blisters or crusting appearing, the client should be advised to refrain from picking the area. Blisters should not be pricked but allowed to dry out naturally. The client should be advised to contact the clinic for advice and reassurance if she or he is at all concerned. The doctor may recommend the used of antibiotics in some instances.

Side effects

It is important that clients have not exposed their skin to the sunlight for at least a month before treatment. This may cause the skin to react by swelling after treatment and increase the possibility of crusting after treatment. Too much sun exposure immediately before or after laser treatment can cause alteration in the pigmentation of the skin, which can take months to subside, and in extreme circumstances cause permanent lightening of the skin.

Contra-indications

- ◆ Exposure to sunlight
- ◆ Pregnancy
- ◆ Anti-coagulants, e.g. warfarin or aspirin
- ◆ Dysmorphobia
- ◆ Diabetes
- ◆ Broken skin surface
- ◆ Haemophilia
- ◆ Asthma.

The registration of establishments using class 3b, 3a and 4 lasers

On 1 April 2002, it became a legal requirement for all establishments using intense pulsed light systems and class 3b lasers and above to register with the National Care Standards. Details of this legislation are given in Chapter 16 page 125.

Summary

Lasers are used to treat a wide range of vascular disorders from facial telangiectasia, spider naevi, port wine stains and strawberry naevi to capillary matting and spider thread veins of the legs.

Lasers emit a fixed wavelength to target a specific chromophore. The aim is to destroy the capillaries or veins by selective photothermolysis.

Laser treatment can be used on its own or in combination with other treatments such as sclerotherapy, short-wave diathermy, blend or intense pulsed light. The choice of treatment will depend on the specific needs of the individual.

100 per cent clearance of veins and capillaries can not be guaranteed. The success rate will depend on many factors, therefore clients should be given realistic expectations of the results – usually between 50–70 per cent clearance. In many instances, clients do have a higher percentage clearance; however, it is better to promise less to avoid disappointment.

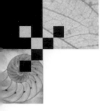

Review questions

1 What are the main differences between intense pulsed light and laser?

2 What does the term 'LASER' mean?

3 Name the lasers that are used for the treatment of facial and/or leg veins.

4 Describe the treatment procedure for facial veins with laser.

5 List the important points of aftercare advice that should be given to clients.

6 Why is it important that clients do not pick at scabs after laser treatment?

7 Describe the appearance of the skin after laser treatment.

8 What is meant by 'selective photothermolysis'?

9 Define the following terms:

   a 'chromophore'

   b 'monochromatic'

   c 'fluence'.

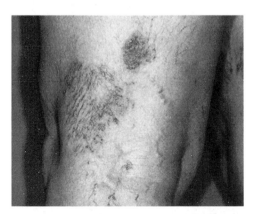 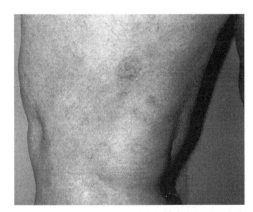

Figure 14.3   Before and after treatment of varicose veins with NdYag laser

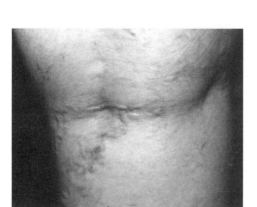
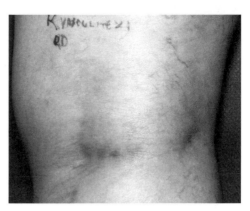

Figure 14.4 Female with varicose and spider veins 3 months after two laser and three IPL treatments

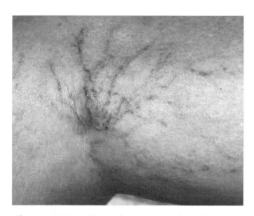
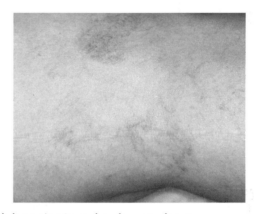

Figure 14.5 Complex networks – female with leg veins 3 weeks after one laser treatment

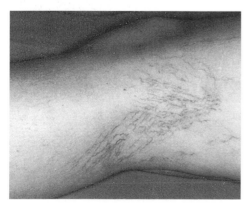
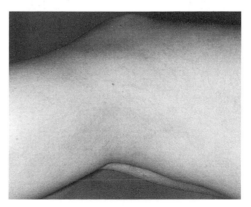

Figure 14.6 Female with complex networks 8 months after one combined laser and IPL treatment

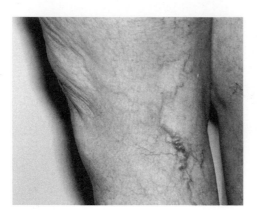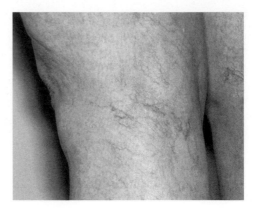

Figure 14.7   Female with varicose veins 6 weeks after one laser treatment

Hygiene and sterilisation

Key points

1 The treatment of telangiectasia by epilation is an invasive procedure.

2 Hepatitis viruses are far more resilient than HIV and are capable of existing for considerable periods of time on infected needles and hard surfaces.

3 Vaccination against hepatitis B is advisable for people working in high-risk occupations.

4 Septicaemia can occur as a result of *needle stick injury*.

5 Needle stick injury is the name given to the accidental piercing of the skin with a needle, e.g. an epilation needle, micro-lance or hypodermic needle.

6 High standards of hygiene must be observed to prevent cross infection.

The treatment of telangiectasia and the removal of minor skin blemishes by electrical epilation is classed as an invasive procedure. During the majority of these procedures, the electrolysist's insertions come into direct contact with blood. Certain procedures may also be responsible for blood seeping onto the skin's surface. It is well known that conditions such as hepatitis, AIDS and septicaemia can all be contracted through direct or indirect contact with contaminated blood or needles. Cases of infection through blood containing HIV or hepatitis during surgery, acupuncture and dental treatment have all been recorded.

Hygiene procedures

Strict adherence to clinical hygiene and sterilisation procedures are essential to protect both the client and the electrolysist. Setting and maintaining strict hygiene routines reduces the risk of cross infection between clients and keeps the risk of infection from the client to the electrolysist, or vice versa, to a minimum. This can easily be achieved in the following ways.

1 All treatment rooms should be cleaned thoroughly on a regular basis: floors, windows, treatment couches, the operator's chair/stool, trolley, machine, magnifying lamp and waste bins should all be included.

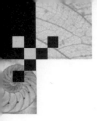

2 Regular cleaning of all equipment and sterilisation of forceps and needles should be implemented.

3 Cuts and abrasions should be covered at all times and disposable gloves used during treatments.

4 Hands should be washed immediately before and after all client contact, and nails should be kept clean by the use of a nail brush.

5 The electrolysist should wear disposable gloves during treatment.

6 Clinic waste should be disposed of correctly and regularly.

Hygiene terms

There are number of terms that the practising electrolysist should be familiar with.

Asepsis: the absence of infection from micro-organisms.

Aseptic: free from organisms capable of causing disease.

Bacteria: small, one-cell, micro-organisms that need a moist warm atmosphere in order to survive. They also need oxygen, and they give out carbon dioxide. Some bacteria are harmless to the human body, e.g. those found in the digestive tract. Others are responsible for conditions such as impetigo, food poisoning and boils.

Bactericide: a chemical agent that will kill most bacteria but is not effective on viruses.

Sepsis: the presence of infection due to micro-organisms.

Sterilisation: the process used to achieve total destruction of all living organisms and spores.

Virus: minute particles that are completely inactive outside the living cells they infect. In suitable environments they are capable of reproduction and mutation (see W.G. Peberdy, *Sterilisation and Hygiene*, 1988). Examples of viral infections are: influenza, the common cold, hepatitis A, B, C, and D, and HIV.

Hygiene in the clinic

Hygiene within the clinic is easily achieved and the procedure should be a routine matter. All equipment, hard work surfaces and washable floors should be wiped over daily with a hospital grade disinfectant. There are many of these available on the market, a number of which are environmentally friendly. Hand washbasins should be cleaned regularly. Soap bars should be placed in a soap rack between use, although soap pump dispensers are more hygienic, and hands should be dried on disposable paper towels.

Disinfectants and sterilisation

When using disinfectants for the purpose of killing viruses and bacterial spores, it is essential that the manufacturer's instructions for dilution percentages are strictly adhered to. Accurate timing of the immersion of objects in disinfectant is important.

The disadvantage of some of the strong disinfectants is the risk of skin irritation or allergies. A few may not be environmentally friendly, which causes a problem when disposing of the solution.

Solutions containing chlorhexidine combine a high level of antibacterial activity with low toxicity and should be used after washing with soap to disinfect the hands prior to giving treatment and preparing the skin for electro-epilation.

The majority of disinfectant and antiseptic preparations have a limited shelf life once they have been made into solution, therefore it is wise to be guided by the manufacturer's recommendations.

Treatment couches should be covered with fresh disposable paper towels for each client. Used clinic waste, such as paper towels, cotton wool swabs, paper tissues and disposable gloves, should be placed in a covered container lined with a plastic bag. The plastic bag should be securely tied and disposed of daily.

Surfaces contaminated by blood should be cleaned using disposable gloves and paper towels, which should then be discarded into a plastic bag.

Containers holding contaminated probes or forceps should be cleaned and sterilised daily. Instruments, which have been dropped on the floor, should be washed and re-sterilised before use.

Needles

Although it is possible to sterilise needles in an autoclave, it is not the ideal solution, being inefficient, time consuming, and therefore not cost effective. With the advent of pre-sterilised disposable needles, the risk of cross infection from inadequately sterilised needles is eliminated. Clients are given peace of mind when they see a new needle being removed from the packet and inserted into the needle holder. It is particularly important with advanced techniques that any risk of cross infection is eliminated due to the invasive nature of the treatment. An innovation to electrolysis is the Probex needle holder. The unique design of this needle holder enables the needle to be loaded easily without risk of damage or contamination as described in the following steps.

1   Remove the Probex needle from the box.

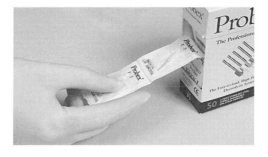

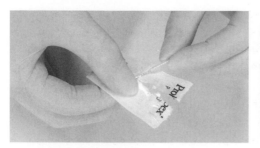

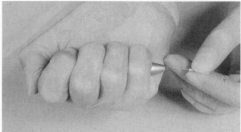

2 Tear the sachet lengthways and remove the needle by holding the protective sleeve.

3 Depress the load mechanism with thumb.

4 Insert the needle into the needle holder jaws until the coloured Steri Guard is flush with the jaws.

5 Release the load mechanism so that the needle is gripped firmly and slide off the protective sleeve.

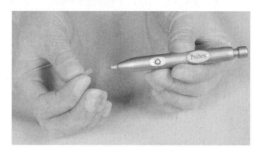

6 After use, hold the needle over the sharps box, depress the load mechanism and allow the needle to drop safely into the box.

Disposable needles are sterilised in one of two ways.

1 Needles are packed in hospital grade blister packs and sterilised with ethylene oxide gas. The expiry date of the needle is stamped on the packet, e.g. Ballet Needles.

2 Individually packed needles are sterilised by gamma irradiation – these packets have a red dot on the outside that proves that sterilisation has taken place, e.g. Sterex and Carlton, or a coloured strip down the side of the packet, e.g. Probex.

After use, needles should be placed directly into the sharps box. Sharps boxes should be disposed of when they are three-quarters full.

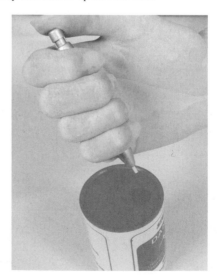

Figure 15.1
Sharps box

Glass bead sterilisers are not recommended for the sterilisation of needles. Attempts to sterilise needles in this way damage the tip of the needle, in addition to which the needle can easily become bent and damaged. The result is that needles are not fit for use and an effective exercise in false economy.

Needle stick injury

Needle stick injury is the name given to the accidental piercing of the skin with a needle, e.g. an epilation needle, a micro-lance or a hypodermic needle. When this occurs with a contaminated needle, it is possible for septicaemia or cross infection with hepatitis or HIV to occur. To prevent needle stick injury, disposable and damaged or bent needles should not be straightened or otherwise manipulated by hand. Instead they should be placed in a puncture resistant container (sharps box) that is securely sealed. The sharps box should be disposed of in the manner specified by the local environmental health office (usually found within council offices).

Needle holders, caps, chucks and forceps

Needle holders should be wiped over with a detergent solution (germicide or disinfectant) after each treatment. Plastic or metal caps, chucks and forceps should be immersed in a disinfectant solution for at least 1 hour, then rinsed in water and dried with tissue or a paper towel prior to use, or cleaned with soap/detergent and water, rinsed and then immersed in 70 per cent isopropyl alcohol for at least 10 minutes. The covered container used to hold the alcohol should be emptied daily or whenever visibly contaminated, whichever applies first. These items may also be cleaned by washing in a bactericidal soap/detergent and rinsing before being placed in a covered solution for 10 minutes.

Forceps, metal caps and chucks are all suitable for sterlisation in the autoclave. These items should be sterilised in the autoclave after each use due to the invasive nature of the treatment.

Disposable materials

Consumables such as cotton wool pads, paper bed roll, tissues (which may have been used to protect the client's eyes against the light, or for the client's personal use when treatment to the nose or upper lip caused a fit of sneezing) and disposable gloves should be discarded into a lined covered container immediately after use. Bin liners should be replaced daily. Sharps boxes containing contaminated needles and micro-lances should be collected by the local Department of the Environment on request, or arrangements should be made with the local hospital.

Hand preparation prior to treatment

The hands should be washed with liquid soap or bactericidal preparations immediately before and after treatment and dried either under a hot air drier or with disposable paper towels.

All cuts, abrasions and open wounds should be covered with a waterproof dressing prior to treatment, and disposable gloves worn throughout the treatment.

A fresh pair of disposable gloves is recommended for every client. These should be changed when damaged. When treatment has been interrupted, gloves should either be washed in bactericidal/germicidal solution or changed for a fresh pair.

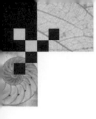

Personal hygiene

The electrolysist's personal hygiene and general appearance give an insight into the character of the individual. Untidy hair, bad breath, soiled uniforms, scuffed shoes, grubby fingernails, aromas such as stale cigarette smoke, yesterday's curry or garlic all create an unfavourable impression. On the other hand, well-groomed hair, short manicured nails without nail polish, clean shoes, a newly laundered uniform and fresh breath all contribute to a smart, well cared for appearance which will not be missed by the clients.

Preparation of skin prior to treatment

All make-up should be removed from the area. Chlorhexidine solution or a spirit swab may be used to wipe the area, after which the cotton wool or swab should be discarded immediately. The skin surface should then be dried with a disposable tissue. If a lignocaine preparation is being used, it should be applied now with the aid of a cotton bud or swab.

Surgical spirit is not recommended due to its flammable nature and drying effect on the skin.

Sterilisation methods

Autoclaves

An autoclave is a piece of equipment which allows certain items such as forceps, metal caps, chucks and scissors to be sterilised by steam at temperatures of 121°C under pressure. Modern autoclaves have thermochromic indicators that change colour when the required temperature has been reached. A stacking system is usually provided so that the items can be placed at different levels. Temperatures range from 121–134°C and with the correct time and heat exposure all spores are killed. However, the temperature range may unfavourably affect some materials.

CIDEX OPA

CIDEX OPA (ortho-phtalaldehyde) is active within 5 minutes and is effective in destroying a wide range of micro-organisms including viruses, bacteria, spores and fungi. The effective life span is 14 days and the shelf life of an unopened bottle is 2 years. Metals and plastic can safely be submerged in CIDEX OPA. The active solution should be tested regularly to ensure that the minimum effective concentration for high level disinfection is still effective. Testing is easily carried out by the use of a CIDEX OPA solution test strip. It is always advisable to read the manufacturer's instructions. Once the solution has come to the end of its useful life, it can be poured down the drain and washed away with plenty of water. It is not harmful to the environment.

Infections and viruses

HIV/AIDS

The full name for AIDS is Acquired Immune Deficiency Syndrome, which develops as a result of infection by the Human Immuno-deficiency Virus (HIV).

The virus can be transmitted by infected blood entering the body through sexual contact, through entry via open wounds, contaminated hypodermic, acupuncture or electro-epilation needles.

A small percentage of cases of infection after blood transfusions from infected donors were recorded in the 1980s.

HIV positive means that the virus is present in the body and over a period of time it will impair the body's defense mechanism by interfering with the immune system. HIV interferes with the immune system to reduce the body's ability to fight disease or infections such as pneumonia or influenza. It is these secondary infections that often prove fatal. A person who is HIV positive may show all or some of the following symptoms:

◆ general fatigue

◆ inability to recover fully from infections such as colds, influenza or pneumonia

◆ enlargement of the lymph nodes

◆ weight loss

◆ diarrhoea.

HIV is a fragile virus when exposed to air, and is one that is easily destroyed by the use of disinfectants.

Hepatitis

The hepatitis A,B,C,D,E,F and G viruses are far more resilient than HIV and are capable of existing for considerable periods of time on infected needles and hard surfaces.

The name 'hepatitis' means 'inflammation of the liver'. There are six categories of virus that cause hepatitis.

1 **Hepatitis type A (HAV):** infective hepatitis, also known as short incubation hepatitis. It is spread by the faecal and oral route. The symptoms are diarrhoea and vomiting.

2 **Hepatitis type B-serum (HBV):** also known as long incubation hepatitis. It affects the liver and is transmitted in the blood.

3 **HCV:** formerly known as non-A and non-B hepatitis. The incubation period is between 20–90 days.

4 **HDV:** also known as hepatitis delta virus. This is the only virus that is known to affect animals as well as humans.

5 **HEV:** discovered in 1990. Transmitted by drinking water infected by contaminated faeces and possibly by blood. As yet, there is no vaccine available.

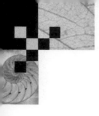

6 **HGV:** also known as GB virus-C, a recently discovered form of hepatitis. Transmitted by exposure to infected blood.

Hepatitis A

Hepatitis A is of short duration with an incubation period of approximately 1 month. This particular virus can be contracted from contaminated food or water. The hepatitis A virus is lost from the body fairly quickly.

Hepatitis B

Hepatitis B is a far more serious condition of longer duration. The incubation period varies from between 40–160 days, during which time the patient is highly infectious. A person infected with hepatitis B feels generally unwell and fatigued for a lengthy period of time, e.g. several months. This is followed by a long convalescence.

Symptoms shown in the early stages include nausea, vomiting, loss of appetite and general fatigue. The whites of the eyes, together with the skin and the gums, may take on a yellow appearance. Fever may also be present in the early stages of infection. Unlike hepatitis A, the B virus remains in the body for a considerable length of time.

Contaminated needles and blood may easily transmit the hepatitis B virus. This virus can also be transmitted through needle stick injury, contact with infected blood, through an open wound, blood transfusion, or drug users sharing needles. It has been found that the virus can remain inactive on hard surfaces for several years, therefore high standards of hygiene in the clinic are imperative.

Vaccination against hepatitis B is possible and advisable for people working in high-risk occupations. The procedure consists of three vaccinations, the first two spaced 1 month apart and the third 6 months later. Details and information can be obtained from the local doctors' surgery.

Hepatitis C

Hepatitis C is blood-borne and lies between A and B in severity. Symptoms, which are similar to those of influenza, are gradual in their onset and are milder than those of hepatitis A and B. The incubation period is between 20–90 days. Hepatitis C carries an increased risk of liver cancer in later life. A vaccine is not available for hepatitis C. Acquisition is through the use of infected syringes, where syringes are used by more than one person as with drug users, through post-blood transfusion and occupational exposure.

Septicaemia

Septicaemia can occur as a result of needle stick injury. Bacteria and toxins are present in the blood. In mild cases the infected area becomes inflamed, swollen, hot and sore to the touch. After a short period of time pus will form. Treatment is by antibiotics.

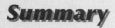

Summary

Advanced electrical epilation is an invasive procedure, more often than not involving direct insertions into blood capillaries. High standards of hygiene must be observed to prevent cross infection.

Diseases such as hepatitis and HIV are easily transmitted through blood. HIV is fragile when exposed to air although hepatitis is far more resilient, being able to survive on hard work surfaces and on needles for a considerable time. The electrolysist can be protected against contracting hepatitis by immunisation and ensuring that disposable gloves are worn during all treatments. Hygiene and sterilisation procedures within the clinic should be a matter of routine.

Review questions

1 Define the following terms:

   a 'hygiene'

   b 'sterilisation'.

2 Why should cuts and abrasions on the skin be covered when practicing advanced electrical epilation?

3 Define the following terms:

   a 'bacteria'

   b 'virus'

   c 'septicaemia'

   d 'sepsis'.

4 Explain the difference between a person who has been diagnosed with AIDS and a person who is HIV positive.

5 What does the term 'hepatitis' mean?

6 Why is it advisable for an electrolysist to be vaccinated against hepatitis B?

7 How can septicaemia and cross infection occur as a result of needle stick injury?

8 Give the two methods that are used to sterilise disposable epilation needles.

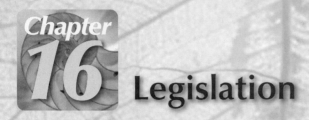

Chapter 16 Legislation

Key points

1 Legislation does not stand still. The electrolysist must ensure that she or he keeps up to date with changes as and when they occur.

2 Electrolysists should be registered with the local Environmental Health Department under the Local Government (Miscellaneous Provisions) Act 1982.

3 Establishments operating lasers and intense pulsed light systems are legally required to register with the National Care Standards Commission in line with the Care Standards Act 2000.

4 Procedures such as risk assessment and COSHH require time and thought to set up initially.

Much of the legislation for the electrolysis profession is basic common sense and is in place to protect the health of the practitioner, the employee and the general public. Ignorance of the law is no excuse when a representative from the local environmental office arrives on the doorstep. An inspector from the Environmental Health Department has the right to call on the clinic/premises at any time without notification. The inspector has the authority to investigate claims of unsafe practice or to follow up a formal complaint that may have been lodged with the department. The inspector will give details of the nature of the complaint, discuss these with the proprietor and will follow this with a written report. Should the complaint be upheld, the inspector has the power to serve an improvement notice that must state the nature of the complaint and the time limit given to rectify the situation. Where the inspector finds that the personal safety of employees or the general public is endangered, he or she has the authority to serve a prohibition notice which requires the employer to cease the unsafe practice immediately and/or face prosecution.

The Environmental Health Department

It is the responsibility of all practicing electrolysists to be registered with the Local Environmental Health Department under The Local Government (Miscellaneous Provisions) Act 1982. It is the operator who must be registered, not the premises. A representative from the Environmental Health Department will visit the premises and communicate with the individual before issuing a certificate of registration.

In addition to the above, the following information relates to some of the main legislation applicable to the business. It is not, however, an exhaustive list.

1   Health and Safety at Work Act 1974

2   Electricity at Work Regulations Act 1989

3   Fire Precautions Act 1971

4   Control of Substances Hazardous to Health Regulations (COSHH) 2003

5   The Management of Health and Safety at Work Regulations 1999

6   The Health and Safety (First Aid) Regulations 1981

7   The Medicines for Human Use (Marketing Authorisations etc.) Regulations 1994 (particularly pertinent for electrolysists using topical anesthetics or practicing sclerotherapy)

8   Working Times Regulations 1998

9   The Care Standards Act 2000

10 Data Protection Act 1998.

Electrical epilation legislation

The Local Government (Miscellaneous Provisions) Act 1982

This Act requires that any person carrying out electrical epilation should be registered with the local authority before commencing practice. Failure to register could result in a fine of up to £200.

The inspector, prior to issuing a registration certificate, will want to know the following information:

◆ provisions for sanitation

◆ hygiene procedures

◆ sterilisation methods for equipment, forceps, chucks, metal caps, etc.

◆ whether or not sterilised disposable needles are used – most local authorities now insist on the use of disposable needles

◆ methods for the disposal of contaminated sharps

◆ storage of used sharps containers whilst awaiting disposal

◆ storage of consumables such as bed rolls, tissues, cotton wool and antiseptic lotions.

Each local authority will draw up their own set of by-laws under section 15(7) of the Local Government (Miscellaneous Provisions) Act 1982. The by-laws may vary from one authority to another.

Section 16(9) of the Act requires the registered person to display a copy of the by-laws and their certificate of registration prominently on the premises.

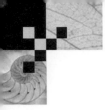

Health and Safety at Work Act 1974

The purpose of this Act is to give protection to employers, employees including contractors, and members of the public. The Act is concerned with the protection of the individual against health and safety risks arising from, or in connection with, the activities of another person at work. The requirements of the Act are far reaching.

The employer must ensure that:

◆ the health, safety and welfare of employees is catered for – this means that the working environment must be maintained at a reasonable working temperature, that ventilation is effective, that lighting is suitable and that there are adequate toilet and washing facilities

◆ there are duties that include the provision of training, instruction and supervision

◆ a safety policy is prepared and reviewed regularly.

The employee is responsible for:

◆ taking reasonable care of her or his health and safety at work by following the health and safety procedures

◆ taking reasonable care of other persons who may be affected by her or his actions or omissions at work

◆ treating all equipment properly and reporting any faults.

Health and Safety Legislation 1992 – the 'six pack'

Under the umbrella of the Health and Safety at Work Act is a set of regulations, commonly referred to as the 'six pack', which was introduced to fulfill European Union Directives. It is formed from six regulations.

1 The Management of Health and Safety at Work Regulations 1999 – a key requirement of these regulations is the need to conduct a risk assessment. An employer with five or more employees will have to record the significant findings of the assessments.

2 The Provision and Use of Work Equipment Regulations 1998 – these regulations are intended to ensure the provision of safe work equipment and its safe use.

3 Manual Handling Operations Regulations 1999.

4 Workplace (Health, Safety and Welfare) Regulations 1992.

5 Personal Protective Equipment at Work (PPE) Regulations 1992 – this is defined as all equipment designed to be worn or held, such as face masks, eye wear and gloves, to protect people against risks to their health and safety.

6 Health and Safety (Display Screen Equipment) Regulations 1992 – these regulations set out the obligations of employers to assess the risks arising out of the use of display screen equipment, which may cause injury at work. Some known problems associated with the use of such equipment include repetitive strain injury, eye strain and headaches.

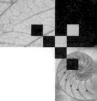

Detailed information relating to the above legislation is available in the reference section of the local library.

Risk assessment

The employer or salon manager is required to carry out *risk assessment* on a regular basis. This involves identifying a risk, assessing the extent of the risk, and taking measures to protect the staff and clients. Potential hazards should be identified and action taken to prevent accidents occurring. Hazards can be described as anything that can cause harm, whereas a risk is the chance, small or large, that an individual will actually be harmed by the hazard.

A risk assessment should include the following points:

◆ identification of the potential hazard

◆ who might be harmed and how

◆ an evaluation of the risk arising from the hazard

◆ a decision as to whether the existing precautions are adequate or whether they should be altered.

Risk assessments should be reviewed regularly and amended when necessary.

Fire Precautions Act 1971

This Act states that all employees should:

◆ be aware and trained in emergency fire evacuation procedures

◆ know where the nearest emergency exits are situated – *these exits must be kept clear at all times during working hours*

◆ be aware of the fact that lifts must not be used in the event of a fire or power failure

◆ be aware that in the event of a fire all personal belongings should be left behind

◆ know that all windows and doors should be closed on leaving the premises wherever possible

◆ be aware of the location of the fire appliances, the type of fire extinguishers, their uses and how to use them

◆ know that consumables such as paper bed rolls, surgical spirits, etc., should be stored well away from any possible risk of fire

◆ know that magnifying lamps should be kept away from direct sunlight – when direct sunlight is concentrated through the lens onto a flammable material, fire may result due to the build up of heat.

Electricity at Work Regulations Act 1989

These regulations require that all electrical equipment be maintained in a safe condition. One way of achieving this is to implement regular checks by a qualified electrician who will then label the equipment stating the date of inspection.

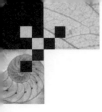

Control of Substances Hazardous to Health (COSHH) 2003

This regulation covers the storing and use of products containing hazardous substances, e.g. surgical spirit, glutaradehyde, chlorhexidine and bleach.

The regulations require that all products containing substances known to present a hazard to health should be subject to an assessment that considers their safe use, first aid measures and details of action to be taken in case of accidental exposure.

(a) Corrosive   **(b) Explosive**   **(c) Harmful**   **(d) Highly flammable**

(e) Irritant   **(f) Oxidizing**   **(g) Toxic**

Figure 16.1
COSHH
symbols

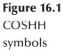

The Medicines Act 1968

The retail sale and supply of medicines is regulated by the Medicines Act 1968. Under the Act, each medicine that is publicly available is assigned to one of three legal categories:

1 Prescription only medicine (POM), which may only be supplied through a pharmacy against a doctor's prescription.

2 Pharmacy medicines (P), which are supplied through a pharmacy under the supervision of a pharmacist.

3 General sales list medicines (GSL), which are available from other retail outlets.

Four anesthetics that are licensed for topical use are:

1 Emla cream 5 per cent (POM)

2 Emla patch 1G (POM)

3 Syntex Ethyl Chloride BP 100 per cent (P)

4 Amnitop.

Electrolysists should note that Emla cream and Emla patch 1G are classed under the Medicines Act as prescription only medicine (POM) and may only be supplied from pharmacies against a doctor's prescription. Therefore, an electrolysist cannot obtain this product for general use when undertaking advanced epilation for the removal of telangiectasia. However, it is perfectly legal for the client's doctor to issue a prescription for the client's personal use immediately prior to or during treatment.

The registration of premises for the use of lasers and intense pulsed light systems

The Care Standards Act 2000 came into force on 1 April 2002. Providers of laser and intense pulsed light treatments are required to register their premises with the National Care Standards Commission. Certain criteria must be met before a registration certificate is issued. This is not an Act that is standing still; a number of changes to the implementation of the Act occurred in September 2003, with further changes to come in the future. It is essential that the owner of a registered establishment and the manager keep up to date with changes as and when they occur.

In England, the Act requires the independent National Care Standards Commission to undertake this regulatory function. In Wales, this function will be carried out by a new section of the National Assembly for Wales, which will be established as either a department or an agency of the National Assembly for Wales.

The Care Standards Act 2000 replaces the Registered Homes Act 1984 (which is to be repealed in its entirety). All establishments that offer laser and intense pulsed light treatments are required by law to be registered with the National Care Standards Commission.

Data Protection Act 1998

Clients are now entitled to ask for copies of any information that has been stored in relation to themselves. Only information of a professional nature should be recorded together with appointments, etc. It is not wise to store any personal observations or comments. Data must not be kept for longer than is necessary and should be updated regularly to ensure that the information held is accurate.

When records containing personal information relating to clients are kept on computer, it is a legal requirement for the user to register with the Data Protection Register.

The law applies to all businesses and records held no matter how small the business is. There are some exceptions to this rule. Failure to register is a criminal offence and can result in a fine of several thousand pounds.

The application forms DPR1 or DPR4 (intended for use by small businesses) are available from:

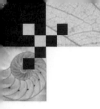

The Data Protection Registrar
Wycliff House
Water Lane
Wilmslow
Cheshire SK9 5AF
www.dataprotection.gov.uk
Tel: 01625 545745

Legislation cannot be ignored and is part of everyday working life. It is the responsibility of the employer and employee to ensure the health and safety of themselves, their colleagues and their clients.

Procedures such as risk assessment and COSHH (Control of Substances Hazardous to Health) require time and thought to set up initially. Once in place, it should become a routine matter to keep these up to date and revised where necessary on a regular basis. Electrolysists are required by law to be registered with the Environmental Health Department of the local council under the Local Government (Miscellaneous Provisions) Act 1982. Practitioners using intense pulsed light and laser systems are required to comply with the conditions of the Care Standards Act 2000, which is governed by the National Care Standards Commission. Establishments that keep computerised records should also register with the Data Protection Register.

Summary

Legislation affects everyone, whether your role is an electrolysist working with the general public, employing staff, or as an employee. There are many pitfalls that need to be avoided. Laws change or new ones are introduced on a regular basis and *it is your responsibility* to ensure that you keep up to date. Ignorance is no excuse in a court of law. The library, Internet, ACAS and Environmental Health Department at your local council are all good sources of information.

Electrolysists should register with the Local Environmental Health Department for the Local Government (Miscellaneous Provisions) Act 1982. Those salons/clinics offering laser and intense pulsed light treatments should also register with The National Care Standards Commission. Remember that there will be changes, which will affect the management of the Care Standards Act 2000, and that it is the responsibility of the clinic manager or owner to keep up to date and be aware of the changes as and when they happen.

In addition to the above two Acts, key legislation includes:

◆ the Health and Safety at Work Act 1974

◆ COSHH regulations 2003

◆ the Health and Safety Legislation 1992 – the safety legislation collectively known as the 'six pack'.

Review questions

1 Name six Acts that electrolysists must comply with.

2 What is the Local Government (Miscellaneous Provisions) Act 1982?

3 List the main points covered in Health and Safety Legislation 1992 – the 'six pack'.

4 What does 'COSHH' stand for?

5 Briefly describe the Medicines Act 1968.

6 What is the purpose of the Data Protection Act 1998?

7 Who should register with the Data Protection Register?

8 Name the governing body for the Care Standards Act 2000.

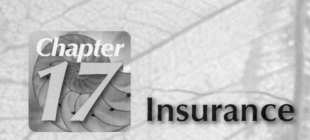

Chapter 17

Insurance

Key points

1 Having the right insurance cover can help to give you peace of mind.

2 Before setting up in practice contact a reputable insurance broker who will be able to advise you on the policies you will need.

3 In the event of a claim, the electrolysist could well be facing financial ruin without the right cover in place, e.g. treatment risk, fire or business interruption.

4 Certain policies are required by law, e.g. employer's liability, public liability.

5 Record cards must be accurate and up to date.

Insurance cover now, more than ever, is essential to the practicing electrolysist. Members of the general public are not so hesitant about taking legal action if they feel they have a grievance. Some claims are justified, whereas others are not. Either way, an electrolysist could suffer more than a few sleepless nights if she or he does not have the correct insurance policy in place, particularly in the event of a successful claim. Without the right insurance cover, the electrolysist could well be facing financial ruin!

Access to legal aid is not as readily accessible as it has been in the past. However, many solicitors now offer a 'No win, no fee' service, which is attractive to claimants. Legal fees are often based on a high percentage of the final settlement. The majority of claims arise as the result of treatment being carried out incorrectly or carelessly. The introduction of pre-sterilised disposable needles has made a difference, with fewer claims made for incorrect hygiene procedures.

Before deciding which insurance company to use, it would be prudent to contact a reputable insurance broker who should be fully conversant with the different policies available. The professional associations should also be able to guide members in the direction of an insurance broker who will be familiar with the electrolysists' needs.

After discussing your specific needs, the insurance broker will be able to advise you on policies that suit your requirements. Before making a final decision, it is essential that the policy is read (including the small print!) and the wording carefully checked. The exact terminology can be very important. The professional associations, such as the British Association of Electrolysists, the Institute of Electrolysis, BABTAC and the Guild, offer optional extensions through their group insurance cover. These professional bodies have stringent conditions with regard to professional qualifications and training, which must be met before members are eligible for cover. The conditions vary between the associations, therefore these must be checked carefully. It is always advisable to check that the insurance company understands what your needs are, so when using an insurance broker, go to one that is fully conversant with the needs of your profession.

The law requires that policies include:

◆ the employer's liability when employing people

◆ car insurance as it may be necessary to insure the car for business purposes dependent on the nature of use

◆ public liability.

Additional policies, which are advisable, include:

◆ treatment risk

◆ product liability

◆ hand disablement

◆ general personal accident

◆ permanent health insurance

◆ salon – buildings and content.

Employer's liability: is a legal requirement when employing staff. It is worth noting that employer's liability will be required even if the only employee is a cleaner or a work experience trainee. This policy covers the employer for legal liability in the event of injury to an employee arising out of their employment. The current certificate should be displayed in a prominent position in the staff room. By law, the employer must keep certificates for a minimum of 40 years.

Car insurance: premiums will be higher when the car is used in connection with business, e.g. mobile therapists. It is necessary to inform the insurance company that cover is required for business use as failure to do so may result in the insurance company refusing to meet any claim that arises when the car is being used for this purpose. It is always worth budgeting for fully comprehensive insurance as opposed to 'Third Party, Fire and Theft'. The extra cost involved will pay for itself if the car is involved in an accident and is seriously damaged, or, even worse, written-off as a result. An additional 'all risks' cover should be taken out for stock and equipment that is carried in the car as these would not be included in the basic policy.

Treatment risk: protects the electrolysist against legal liability for accidental injury to a client arising out of treatment, e.g. scars from incorrect electrical

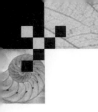

epilation, injury to an eye, or permanent injury, which may result in psychological distress. The onus is on the client to prove that the injury or damage suffered is due to the fault of the electrolysist. However, there are times when the court has to decide on the balance of probabilities – usually in the client's favour! Most cases are settled out of court.

Permanent health insurance: provides long-term protection for loss of income arising though illness, injury or accident. When self-employed, illness or permanent disability can result in serious financial hardship. Financial commitments such as a mortgage, the community charge, electricity, gas, telephone and food bills still have to be met.

Statutory Sick Pay, Sickness Benefit and Invalidity Benefit provided by the government are designed only to protect against poverty and do not provide sufficient income to maintain standards of living. The premiums for permanent health insurance will vary depending on the amount of benefit required, whether there is a deferment period before benefit may be claimed, and the general state of health of the person insured.

Building and contents: main features are protection against the following:

◆ fire, explosion, lightning and earthquake

◆ storm or flood

◆ escape of water from any tank, apparatus or pipe

◆ riot or civil commotion

◆ malicious damage

◆ impact

◆ theft by forcible entry or threat of violence.

The above are just some of the items covered. There may be differences between insurance companies, therefore the policy must be read carefully before making a final decision.

In the event of an insurance claim . . .

What should the electrolysist do when a client indicates that he or she intends to make a claim for injuries received?

◆ Refer to the policy and follow the policy procedure.

◆ Contact the insurance broker as soon as a client indicates her or his intention to make a claim – initial contact to the insurance broker should be by telephone, which should be followed immediately with written confirmation of the name of the claimant, the nature of the claim and the date to which the claim relates.

◆ Any correspondence received from the claimant or claimant's representative should be passed on to the insurance company as soon as possible.

◆ The electrolysist should then gather all relevant documentation relating to the events leading up to the claim.

◆ The electrolysist should not admit liability or get into direct correspondence with the claimant – this is when a photographic record could well be an asset.

Client records

Records are important and must be kept. They should be accurate, detailed, honest and signed; furthermore, they should be kept for at least 6 years. It is very easy to get into the habit or writing the bare essentials on record cards, particularly during very busy periods. However, in the event of an insurance claim, the information provided on the client's record card may be insufficient for the purposes of a court of law.

Clients' record cards should contain the following information:

◆ details of the client's medical history

◆ details of previous treatment by any other electrolysist – if scarring is present, this should be tactfully pointed out to the client during the initial consultation and the location and nature of the scars entered onto the record card together with the date and the client's signature of confirmation. A dated photograph also provides an excellent record

◆ the type and size of the epilation needle should be noted, stating whether it is disposable and pre-sterilised

◆ details of the treatment site, e.g. nose or cheeks

◆ the exact length of the treatment, e.g. 5 minutes, 10 minutes, etc.

◆ current intensity

◆ method used, e.g. short-wave diathermy or blend

◆ the skin's reaction to treatment, e.g. erythema, coagulation – effective or not

◆ the skin's appearance immediately after treatment

◆ if treatment was discontinued for any reason – state the reason

◆ the date of each treatment

◆ advice given to the client with regard to aftercare – N.B. written aftercare instructions should be given to clients at the time of the initial consultation, and the client's signature should be obtained confirming that she or he has received and understood them.

On subsequent visits, prior to giving further treatment, examine the area previously treated and check with the client as to the skin's healing rate after the last appointment. Any abnormal reaction or excessive scabbing should be noted on the client's record card. If the healing rate was slower than anticipated, the client should be questioned, tactfully, as to the aftercare routine to ensure that it has been carried out correctly. It is advisable to ask the client to sign for receipt of the aftercare instructions.

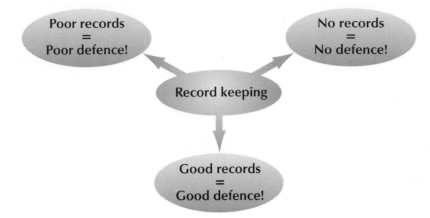

Figure 17.1
Record
keeping

Computerised records

Many electrolysists now keep their client records and appointment system on computer. When this is the case, it is essential to keep a hard copy, which has been signed and dated by the client. These records should be kept up to date with clients signing and dating the records as and when changes occur. Computerised records alone are not acceptable as evidence in a court of law due to the fact that computer records can be altered easily.

The computer should be backed up at the end of each working day. Ideally, two back-up disks should be created. These disks should not be kept with the computer. It is advisable to keep an up-to-date back-up of the computer records at home. In the event of a fire, or flood damage, the records can soon be re-installed thanks to the spare copy.

The legal requirement to register under the Data Protection Act 1998 should not be overlooked (see Chapter 16 page 125).

Doctor's letter

There are certain instances where it is advisable for the electrolysist to ask the client to obtain her or his doctor's agreement prior to treatment being carried out. There are also instances when the insurance company requires the electrolysist to contact the client's doctor before commencing treatment, e.g. moles, warts, etc. Many conditions have similarities with one another and sometimes it can be difficult to distinguish one condition from another.

The aim when contacting a doctor is to keep the letter simple, clear and concise. Doctor's may well charge their patient for writing a letter of agreement. Valuable time can be saved for the doctor by ensuring that the electrolysist's letter contains a section at the end for the doctor's comments and signature. For the doctor's benefit, it is advisable to attach a brief description of the treatment procedure. There are some doctors who may not be familiar with treatment procedure. This letter should then be kept with the client's record card. A sample letter is shown opposite.

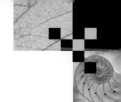

Your name
Address
Postcode
Tel. no.

Ref:

Date

Doctor's Name
Address
Postcode

Dear Dr ....

Re: Patient's name
        Address

Mrs X has been to see me in connection with the removal of
.... on (insert treatment site).
Before I proceed with treatment by short-wave diathermy, would you
be kind enough to examine the area and advise on suitability or any
objections you may have.

Should you have any queries or require further information relating to
treatment, I can be contacted on the above telephone number.

Yours sincerely

Mrs S. Godfrey F.B.A.E., F.I.E., D.R.E., BABTAC
Proprietor
The Sheila Godfrey Clinic

....
Doctor's comments:

I do/do not consent to (patient's name) receiving treatment by
electro-epilation.

Signature:

Date:

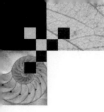

Summary

Now, more than ever, insurance cover for treatment risk is essential. Television adverts often encourage members of the general public to take legal action when they have been involved in an accident or received an injury, on a 'No win – no fee' basis. There is no doubt that sometimes there is cause for such action. However, there are also many instances of individuals intending to sue in order to claim a healthy financial settlement.

During the past few years there has been an increase in loss of business and damage to property due to flood damage in many parts of England and Wales. It is very easy to think 'this will never happen to me', or that such situations 'only affect other people'.

There are a number of insurance policies that can be taken out although some are higher on the priority list than others. Some, such as employer's liability and car insurance are legal requirements.

The practicing electrolysist will also need treatment risk and public liability, although building, contents and business interruption should not be overlooked.

In the event of a client making an insurance claim, the electrolysist should immediately contact the insurance broker and give all the information relating to the situation. This information should include: full details of the incident or treatment, the date, the location, any relevant photographic evidence and a copy of the client's record card. All correspondence received from the client should immediately be passed on to the insurance broker. Do not be tempted to get into detailed discussions with the client or admit responsibility. The insurance company will take over and deal with the situation.

There are instances when it is advisable to contact the client's doctor before commencing treatment. The letter should be kept short and to the point. Where necessary, include a brief description of the treatment involved.

Review questions

1 List the benefits of taking out insurance cover.

2 List five types of insurance cover.

3 Explain the benefits of taking before and after photographs when giving treatment.

4 Why is it necessary to keep accurate and up-to-date records for all clients?

5 Why should any person who keeps computerised records be registered with the Data Protection Register?

6 List the details that should be included on the client's record card.

7 What action should the electrolysist take if a client decides to make an insurance claim against the clinic or practitioner?

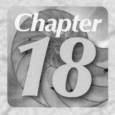

Professional ethics

Key points

1 The term *'professional ethics'* refers to the code of conduct or standards of behaviour practised by the professional electrolysist.

2 It is essential that an electrolysist knows when to refer clients to the medical profession. Equally, busy doctors soon become irritated by unnecessary communication on irrelevant matters.

3 The Institute of Electrolysists Ltd and the British Association of Electrolysists Ltd are the two specialist professional bodies in the UK concerned with epilation.

4 Clients' appointments, once made, should not be cancelled or altered by the electrolysist or their receptionist without good reason.

'Professional ethics' refers to the code of conduct or standards of behaviour practised by the professional electrolysist in relation to:

◆ clients

◆ colleagues

◆ the medical profession

◆ the professional association of which the electrolysist is a member.

Courtesy, honesty and integrity are all essential qualities that separate the caring professionals from the 'cowboys'.

Ethics concerning clients

At all times clients should receive caring, professional treatment. Honest information should be given in relation to the duration and progress of treatment. False promises, or prolonged treatment for financial gain are not beneficial to the electrolysist's long-term reputation. Clients should be given realistic expectations with regard to both short-term and long-term results of treatment, e.g. clients should be advised at the beginning of treatment that it may not be possible to clear large areas of telangiectasia completely, but that instead it may be possible to achieve a reduction of between 60–80 per cent.

The client *must* be able to expect and receive total confidentiality at all times. Information concerning one client should *not* be discussed with another. Conversations involving controversial subjects such as religion, politics and racial matters are best avoided.

Clients' appointments, once made, should not be cancelled or altered by the electrolysist without good reason. There are times when an event such as illness, a death in the family, failure of the electricity supply or a major crisis may prevent the electrolysist from keeping appointments. In such instances the clients must be notified in advance to prevent wasted journeys and possible ill feeling. The majority of clients are very understanding in such circumstances.

The appointment book should be organised to allow for accurate time keeping so that clients are not kept waiting. Running late occasionally is acceptable and inevitable but to do so on a regular basis shows inefficient organisation and a lack of courtesy towards the client.

Many clients are inclined to talk about their personal problems during treatment. The electrolysist is often the only person they can talk to about such matters. It is essential that any conversation takes place in total confidence and is *never* discussed with a third party. In these circumstances the electrolysist should not offer personal advice, since this could give rise to a number of difficulties at a later date. The client's best interests should always be of prime consideration.

Ethics concerning colleagues

A true professional does not attempt to poach clients from colleagues and does not speak disparagingly about another electrolysist's standard of work.

Occasions can arise when an electrolysist will attend to a colleague's clients on a temporary basis, e.g. during holiday periods or times of ill-health. When this situation occurs, the original treatment plan should not be altered in any way without consultation with the colleague concerned.

A minority of clients exist who tend to flit from one clinic to another, or who make appointments with two electrolysists. Once this situation has been brought to the attention of either operator, it must not be allowed to continue, in order to safeguard the electrolysists concerned and to prevent over treatment of the client's skin which may inadvertently result in scarring. Such situations prevent accurate record keeping of treatment progress.

Ethics concerning the medical profession

Clients expect electrolysists to be able to recognise and pass an opinion on any number of skin conditions and medically related matters. It is well known that many skin lesions demonstrate similar characteristics, some of which may be benign, whereas others may be malignant, but this is not for the electrolysist to diagnose. Electrolysists should only provide an opinion on subjects in which they are professionally qualified. There will be times when treatment should not be given without first obtaining written agreement from the client's doctor (see Chapter 17).

The electrolysist's electro-epilation treatments can be divided into three categories: (i) those which cover cosmetic purposes, (ii) those which are hormone related but do not require medical liaison, e.g. the menopause, and (iii) those for which medical referral is advisable, e.g. pigmented naevi.

The initial consultation may indicate the possible existence of a condition that requires medical investigation prior to electro-epilation, e.g. moles or papules that do not heal, or an established disorder such as diabetes. In such circumstances consultation with the client's GP will be necessary before any treatment can be given.

It is essential that the electrolysist knows when to refer clients to the medical profession. Equally, busy doctors soon become irritated by unnecessary communication on irrelevant matters. When a medical practitioner agrees to electro-epilation treatment, progress reports can be sent to that practitioner as and when necessary. This not only keeps the doctor informed but also helps to build a good working relationship between the medical and electrolysis professions.

Professional associations

The two main professional associations in the UK that specialise in electro-epilation are:

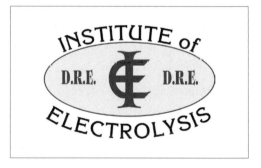

- The British Association of Electrolysists Ltd
- The Institute of Electrolysis Ltd.

Both organisations have similar aims and objectives, which are primarily concerned with promoting the professional status of electrolysis.

Membership of both associations is by examination only. The prospective member is required to demonstrate practical skills in electrolysis and complete a written paper and oral examination. Only when the required standard is achieved is membership to the professional body granted.

Members are required to have gained extensive postgraduate experience in basic epilation techniques before progressing to training in advanced techniques for the removal of telangiectasia etc. Before being entered on the Association's advanced practitioners list, members are required to demonstrate their standards of treatment to a board of examiners.

Membership of a professional body provides many advantages, especially for the electrolysist who works alone in private practice, as individuals are able to keep in touch with other members who work in the same field. Lecture programmes, conferences and annual meetings are arranged for members, which provide excellent ways to keep up to date with any changes in working practice or legal requirements as they take place. Prospective clients often contact a professional association for the name of the nearest electrolysist.

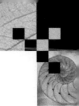

Summary

The electrolysist should conduct herself or himself in a professional manner at all times. She or he should be courteous, considerate and honest towards colleagues, clients, medical practitioners and their professional associations.

Clients should feel confident that they will receive treatment to a high standard and with their best interests in mind.

Review questions

1 Define the term 'professional ethics'.

2 Explain the meaning of 'professional ethics' relating to:

   a clients

   b colleagues

   c the medical profession.

3 List the three categories of electro-epilation treatment covered by an electrolysist.

4 Name the two professional bodies in Britain that specialise in electrical epilation.

5 List the benefits of belonging to a specialist professional body.

Chapter 19

Case studies

Case Study
Client 1: consultation and short-wave diathermy treatment

Sue was an active 35 year old who spent a lot of time outdoors in all weathers. She had a very noticeable spider naevi on the side of the nose and several others, not quite so noticeable, on the cheeks. The main naevus had previously been treated several times in the dermatology department of the local hospital.

The consultation revealed that Sue was a smoker, that she suffered from arthritis, was an advocate of complimentary therapies, and that both her sister and her mother suffered with telangiectasia, spider naevi and skin tags. Sue was given advice on the correct skincare routine that she should follow in order to gain the best results from her treatment.

The treatment application for short-wave diathermy, and its anticipated results were explained to Sue prior to conducting a patch test on one of the smaller spider naevi. An honest and realistic opinion was given with regard to the number of treatments that would be needed. Sue was advised that in view of her family history and the nature of her telangiectasia and spider naevi, the results would not be permanent. She would need to return intermittently. Home care and aftercare were then discussed in detail, and written aftercare instructions were handed to Sue, before she left the clinic, to read at home.

Sue returned to the clinic 4 weeks later. The result of the patch test was good so a full treatment was carried out during this appointment. The appointment session was kept to 15 minutes, with several spider naevi and telangiectasia removed. A gold Tel 4 needle was used (gold is a good conductor of current so a slightly lower intensity can be used). Attention was paid to current intensity and the skin was observed carefully throughout the treatment, with care taken to ensure that treatment was not concentrated in too small an area.

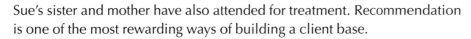

Sue's sister and mother have also attended for treatment. Recommendation is one of the most rewarding ways of building a client base.

The initial course of treatment consisted of five treatments with 4 weeks in between each session. The client was happy with this arrangement. Twenty years later she still returns, spasmodically as the need arises.

A treatment plan for this client is provided for reference on page 142.

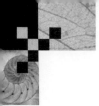

Treatment plan	
Treatment site:	Nose and cheeks
Vascular malformation:	Spider naevi
Method of treatment:	Short-wave diathermy
Needle:	Ballet Tel 4 Gold
Skin reaction:	Naevus blanched immediately, erythema at treatment site. Oedema where needle was inserted. Very small scabs appeared, similar in appearance to a bramble scratch. Scabs fell off during the next 6 days
Appearance of skin following treatment:	Initially the naevi disappeared, then gradually reappeared. The colour became darker over the following 3 days, gradually fading to nothing over the following 3 weeks
Frequency of treatment:	One every 4 weeks
Number of treatments in initial course:	Five
Follow-up appointments:	Spasmodically, as and when required, over a 20-year span

Case study
Client 2: what went wrong?

What went wrong?	
Consultation:	Revealed sensitive skin, telangiectasia to both cheeks, fine texture, October 1986
Medical history:	No contra-indications or medication
Client profile:	Prior to treatment, this lady was outgoing, extrovert, ran the local post office and village shop. Enjoyed meeting people. After treatment she became introvert, lacking in self-confidence, would not socialise and would not work in the post office/shop
Reason for telangiectasia:	Hereditary
Needle size:	Not stated on records
Treatment plan:	One session of 1 hour duration
Reaction to treatment:	Erythema, oedema, pit marks, scabs, tenting of skin, hypo-pigmentation where the needle had been inserted
Client feedback:	Very distressed – took legal action against therapist
Home care advice:	Lavender based aftercare cream

The above table gives an overview of a true event. The lady concerned, Jenny, was a lively, extroverted person who enjoyed socialising and meeting people. Her husband had booked the holiday of a lifetime early in the new year to celebrate her 40th birthday.

During the preceding October, Jenny decided that she would like to get rid of unwanted facial veins. Initially, she attended a reputable establishment in Leeds. The electrolysist gave her a full and detailed consultation, followed by a patch test to see how the skin would react, and also to give her an idea of how the treatment would feel as well as the healing time required after treatment. The electrolysist recommended 5–6 treatments, spaced 4–6 weeks apart. The frequency of the treatments would depend upon the skin's recovery time.

The client could not drive and the trip to Leeds necessitated a 1 hour bus journey. Jenny was therefore delighted to find that the treatment was available at her local beauty salon. Here is where the problems began . . .

The electrolysist at Jenny's local beauty salon had only qualified in basic epilation 8 months previously, having trained in advanced epilation 6 months after completion of the original course.

The client was given a consultation by this young, inexperienced electrolysist who confidently claimed that the treatment could be carried out there and then. The inexperienced electrolysist proceeded to give a 60-minute session to the face and had advised Jenny that only one treatment would be necessary.

The current intensity was too high, causing tenting of the skin and blisters. The size and type of the needle was not recorded. A number of the insertions were too deep – thereby destroying the underlying skin tissue. The long-term result of this was the formation of pit mark depressions in the skin. The needle insertions were also too close together. There was an excessive build-up of heat in the skin and swelling (oedema), which left the skin feeling as if it had been sunburnt. Scabbing was still present on the skin in May of the following year!

The written aftercare instructions and aftercare cream were good. However, due to the incorrect technique and over treatment to the area, Jenny was left with permanent scarring, which could not be camouflaged with make-up. She became introvert and lacking in confidence. Her special birthday party and the longed for holiday were both cancelled.

The moral of this case history is: learn to walk before you run or, to put it another way, be sure that you really are confident with basic epilation for hair removal before taking the next step. A minimum 2 years of continuous clinic or salon experience in epilation for hair removal should be gained before considering training in the advanced techniques.

Case study
Client 3: telangiectasia treatment with blend

Caroline, a 35-year-old lady, lived in a country village in Gloucestershire where she enjoyed horse riding and exercising her dogs. She and her husband had a very busy social life. They travelled extensively – skiing during the winter, and also enjoying holidays in Barbados.

Caroline's skin was dry and sun damaged with pigmentation marks, as well as thread veins around the nose and on both cheeks. Fine lines and wrinkles were present around the eyes and the upper lip.

A treatment plan was drawn up after a detailed consultation and medical history. The number of telangiectasia present suggested that four treatments spaced at four weekly intervals would achieve total clearance of the existing problem. Caroline was advised that the problem may reoccur in time, bearing in mind her lifestyle and the amount of time she spent outdoors.

Caroline received four treatments with blend during each session. The needle used was Tel 3. The appointment sessions were booked for 30 minutes, although the application time for treatment was no more than 10 minutes in total per session.

Caroline was very satisfied with the results of the initial course of treatment. She now attends for the occasional treatment approximately every 3–4 years.

Case study
Client 4: telangiectasia treatment options

A male company director indicated during his initial consultation that he was concerned about the appearance of telangiectasia on his cheeks and around his nose. Aged 45 years, he led an active business life, which involved regular travel abroad. This involved constant flying, changes in temperature from one country to another, changes in time zones, and high levels of stress.

The skin was dry and telangiectasia were present in a rosacea pattern. The client had a very low pain threshold and found it difficult to relax. He held a private pilot's license and enjoyed flying his plane at the weekends. His other hobbies included: sailing, skiing, and driving an open-topped sports car – weather permitting.

There were several treatment options for this client. All of these options, which included laser, IPL, short-wave diathermy and blend, were discussed.

Intense pulsed light was rejected due to the fact that this client often had active pigment in the skin as a result of his lifestyle. Laser was also rejected because the client was not happy about the length of time needed for the skin to recover after treatment. He was not prepared to accept the unsightly appearance of the skin after treatment and during the recovery period.

This client continues to attend for treatment spasmodically as new telangiectasia develop. He usually has a course of between four and six treatments, which keep the skin relatively free of telangiectasia for approximately 2–3 years.

Treatment plan	
Method:	Blend epilation
Frequency of treatments:	One every 4 weeks
Duration of treatment:	10 minutes
Needle:	Ballet Tel 4 Gold
Aftercare:	Aloe vera gel
Skin reaction:	Erythema, lasting approx 2 hours, oedema around the needle insertion, sensation of mild sunburn
Appearance of telangiectasia:	Blanched and disappeared during current application
Appearance of skin following treatment:	During the days following treatment, the telangiectasia appeared to get darker (this is due to the coagulated blood present in the veins); The colour gradually faded during the following 3 weeks
Number of treatments required:	Initial course of six

Case study
Client 5: telangiectasia treatment with short-wave diathermy

This client originally came to the clinic for treatment when she was 22 years old. She has fine, white, delicate skin. Both of her parents were Irish and she had typical Irish colouring, being red hair and fair skin. There were noticeable telangiectasia on both cheeks. The skin flushed easily after hot food, during hot weather, and exposure to sunlight.

A course of five treatments with short-wave diathermy was given, with appointments spaced 6 weeks apart. The appointments were booked for 15 minutes only, due to the sensitivity of the skin. Erythema and oedema were present immediately after each treatment. The oedema usually lasted for approximately 3 days, with the erythema lasting just a few hours. The skin sensation was similar to a very mild sunburn – this was alleviated by the use of cool aloe vera gel after treatment. A stainless steel, flexible two-piece size 4 needle was used.

Case study
Client 6: epilation treatment with blend and IPL

This client, a 58-year-old nurse, initially received six treatments; two with short-wave diathermy followed by four with blend. There were a substantial number of noticeable bluish red veins on both cheeks and around the sides of the nose. There was also an underlying flushing/erythema.

The client works full time, yet finds plenty of opportunity to enjoy her hobbies, which include gardening, playing golf and running (including the London Marathon). Being aware of the increased incidence of skin cancer, this lady was very particular about using a total sunblock on her skin whenever she was outdoors.

The facial capillaries were present over the nose and on both cheeks. The number of capillaries meant that treatment with blend or short-wave diathermy would take place over an 18-month period.

Emla cream was applied to the treatment site 1 hour before treatment as the client found the treatment painful. Her skin was extremely sensitive and her pain threshold was low. Treatment sessions were kept to a maximum of 10 minutes with plenty of healing space allowed between insertions. A gold Tel 3 needle was used. The blend method resulted in less skin trauma. The client also found that blend was more comfortable and the skin healed more quickly after treatment. Appointments were booked 8 weeks apart.

Epilation was followed with two sessions of intense pulsed light to remove the general erythema that gave the client permanent red/rosy cheeks. The two sessions were spaced 8 weeks apart. Erythema and oedema were present immediately after the treatment. The swelling reduced within 5 days and the erythema lasted approximately 4 hours after the first treatment and 3 hours after the second. The capillaries appeared darker immediately after both treatments, gradually fading over the next 3 weeks. The client was delighted with the result.

As with epilation, a patch test was carried out on the treatment site and the results assessed before the full treatment was given.

The following exercises are intended to encourage you to think about:

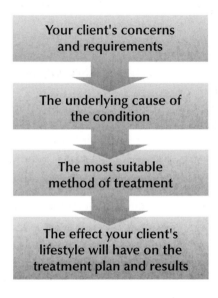

Figure 20.1

Exercises

Exercise 1

Observation of the skin should give you an insight into your client's health and lifestyle. On a blank sheet of paper list the features that you would be looking for and explain how each reflects:

- ◆ health
- ◆ lifestyle.

Explain how the information obtained from the above would influence your:

- ◆ advice and recommendations to your client
- ◆ the treatment plan
- ◆ method of treatment
- ◆ home care recommendations.

Exercise 2

Compare and contrast the skin conditions acne vulgaris and rosacea. State which condition would benefit from electrical epilation and explain why. What would your treatment plan be?

How would the treatment plan for this condition differ from a treatment plan for telangiectasia on the face?

Exercise 3

A client attends the salon with a pale brown mark on the side of the face. This mark appeared shortly after a mole had been removed from the area by laser. What questions would you ask this client? Would you refer this client to a dermatologist for a second opinion? Explain your decision.

Exercise 4

This client is very nervous and lacking in self-confidence. It has taken her 2 years to work up the courage to come into your salon. Her concerns are telangiectasia on the cheeks and nose, also three skin tags on the neck. How would you conduct the initial consultation so that:

1 You help this client to relax.
2 You build her confidence in you.
3 You put her mind at rest with regard to the treatment procedure.

Exercise 5

A number of skin lesions have similar characteristics and appearance. Some are benign and some are malignant. What questions would you ask your client to help you with identification? Describe how you would make an assessment using the ABCD rule given in Chapter 4.

Exercise 6

A 50-year-old lady comes into the salon. Her concerns are telangiectasia to the sides of the nose and a few on the left cheek. She also has spider thread veins and capillary matting on the legs. Draw up a consultation for her and a medical history questionnaire. You will also need to design 'an informed consent to treat' form. Explain which methods of treatment would be suitable and develop a treatment plan. Give reasons for your actions.

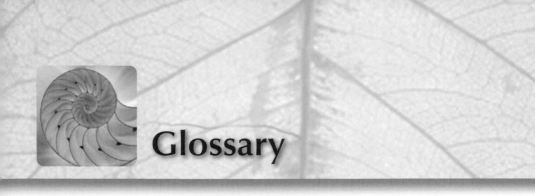

Glossary

Acid mantle   fine film of sebum and sweat found on the surface of the skin.

AIDS   Acquired Immune Deficiency Syndrome, which develops as a result of infection by the Human Immunodeficiency Virus.

Anaphylaxis   (anaphylactic shock) severe allergic reaction to a specific substance that occurs rapidly and in extreme situations may lead to death. The most widely known allergen associated with anaphylaxis is peanuts.

Arterioles   connect arteries to capillaries. The structure is similar to that of arteries but the walls are much thinner.

Artery   strong muscular tube which, with the exception of the pulmonary artery, carries oxygenated blood, hormones, nutrients and other substances.

Benign   non-cancerous, not harmful or invasive.

Capillaries   arterioles gradually reduce in size to form capillaries. Capillaries connect arterioles to venules.

Chromaphore   the light absorbing target in laser and IPL, e.g. melanin in hair removal and haemoglobin in the blood.

Coherence   defined as light waves that are spatially and temporally in phase with one another, i.e. travels in parallel waves with the distance of each peak being exactly the same distance apart.

Collimated   waves of light are emitted in parallel, without divergence as the beam travels through space, e.g. rows of soldiers moving in straight columns in an organised manner, i.e. in parallel to one another.

Contra-indications   presence of a condition that indicates (shows that) treatment should not be given (contra – against).

Dermatofibroma   firm round nodule connected firmly to the epidermis but freely mobile over underlying structures. The colour varies from one lesion to another.

Dysmorphic	refers to a person who will not accept that a particular condition has improved after treatment. As soon as one problem has been resolved, the dysmorphic person will find another that they are convinced has arisen as a result of the original treatment.
Fluence	is the amount of energy delivered to a unit area in a single pulse and is measured in joules or watts per centimetre squared.
Haemangioma	benign tumour composed of vascular tissue.
HIV	Human Immuno-deficiency Virus, which interferes with the body's immune system thereby reducing its ability to fight infection or disease.
Hyper-pigmentation	increased pigmentation. This is often present as a result of sun damage or can occur after treatment by intense pulsed light, laser, short-wave diathermy or sclerotherapy.
Hypo-pigmentation	loss of pigmentation. This can occur as a result of treatment by intense pulsed light, laser or short-wave diathermy.
Intense pulsed light (IPL)	Intense pulsed light is a white, non-coherent, polychromatic light source of variable wavelengths.
Laser	light amplification by stimulated emission of radiation.
Monochromatic	refers to the ability of the laser energy to emit light as a single colour expressed as a wavelength, i.e. blue, orange, yellow, green, red.
Natural moisturising factor	helps to protect against epidermal moisture loss.
Nerve fatigue	when treatment is applied to a specific area for a period of time, e.g. upper lip, nerve endings often respond less efficiently or stop all together. As a result, the client experiences less discomfort.
Perforating vein	connects a superficial vein to a deep vein.
Poikiloderma	patches of blotchy, reddish brown hyper-pigmentation or hypo-pigmentation and telangiectasia. Poikiloderma is found on the neck and is usually associated with sun damage.
POM	Prescription only medicine.
Professional ethics	refers to the code of conduct or standards of behaviour by a professional.
Psoriasis	chronic inflammatory condition of the skin, recognised by well-defined red plaques, which may vary in shape and size, covered with white silver scales.

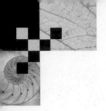

Pulse duration refers to the length of time the laser light is on the tissue.

Reticular vein these veins are often to be seen 'feeding' a patch of veins and are cyanotic to blue in colour.

Sclerosing fluid chemical irritant which has the effect of irritating the walls of the vein, causing it to become inflamed, swollen, then thrombosed.

Sclerotherapy a sclerosing fluid is injected into the vein to bring about the collapse (destruction) of the specific vein.

Spider naevus/naevi central capillary from which fine capillaries radiate – giving the appearance of a spider's legs.

Subdermal plexus is found at the junction of the dermis and subcutaneous layers, and connects freely with the subpapillary layer found in the upper dermis.

Telangiectasia medical term for dilated capillaries. The Greek word telangiectasia means 'end vessel dilation'. Commonly referred to as red veins, broken capillaries or thread veins.

Vein similar in structure to an artery but the walls are thinner, less muscular and contain valves to prevent the backward flow of blood.

Wavelength the colour of light is described by its wavelength. The visible light spectrum ranges from 400 nm, which is blue, to 700 nm, which is red.

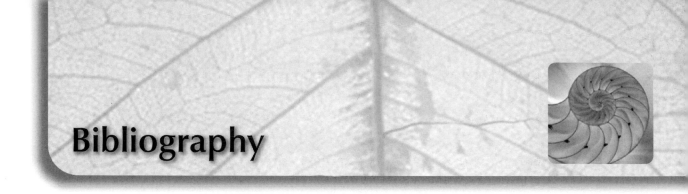

Bibliography

Bennet, R. 1990, *The Science of Beauty Therapy*, London: Hodder & Stoughton

Bono, M. 1991, *The Treatment of Telangiectasia with Blend*, California: Tortoise Press

British Red Cross Society, St John Ambulance and St Andrew's Ambulance Association. 2002, *First Aid Manual*, 8th Edition, London: Dorling Kindersley

Dugge, R.J. 1996, *Anatomy of the Skin*, Connecticut: Internet Dermatology Society

Godfrey, S. 2001, *The Principles and Practice of Electrical Epilation*, 3rd Edition, Oxford: Butterworth Heinemann

Graham-Brown, R. and Burns, T. 2002, *Lecture Notes on Dermatology*, 8th Edition, Oxford: Blackwell Publishers

Gray, H. 1991, *Gray's Anatomy: The Classic Collector's Edition*, New York: Bounty

Hall-Smith, P., Cairns, R.I. and Beare, R.L.B. 1973, *Dermatology*, 2nd Edition, London: Crosby Loickwood Staples

HSE. 2003, COSHH: *A Brief Guide to the Regulations*, Sudbury: HSE Books

HSE. 1998, *Five Steps to Risk Assessment*, Sudbury: HSE Books

HSE. 1994, *Maintaining Portable Electrical Equipment in Offices*, Sudbury: HSE Books

Kirby, J.D. 1986, *Roxburgh's Common Skin Diseases*, 15th Edition, London: H.K. Lewis & Co

Lannigan, S.W. 2000, *Lasers in Dermatology*, London: Springer Verlag UK

Lumines, 2001, *Vasculite Training Manual*, Israel: Lumines Training Manual

MacKie, R.M. 1997, *Clinical Dermatology*, 4th Edition, Oxford: Oxford Medical Publications

Mernagh-Ward, D. and Cartwright, J. 1997, *Good Practice in Salon Management*, Cheltenham: Nelson Thornes

Mernagh-Ward, D. and Cartwright, J. 1997, *Health and Beauty Therapy: A Practical Approach for NVQ Level 3*, 2nd Edition, Cheltenham: Nelson Thornes

Office of the Data Protection Registrar, 1994, *Data Protection Act 1984: The Guidelines*, 3rd Series

Raymond, Dr. E. 2000, *Skin Laser Technology: Application and Treatment*, Loughborough: Loughborough College

Rostein, H. 1993, *Principles and Practice of Dermatology*, 3rd Edition, Oxford: Butterworth Heinemann

Roxburgh, A.C. 2003, *Roxburgh's Common Skin Diseases*, 17th Edition, London: Hodder Arnold

Simmons, J.V. 1989, *The Science of Cosmetics*, London: Macmillan

Vitlae-Lewis, V. 1995, *Sclerotherapy of Spider Veins*, Oxford: Butterworth Heinemann

Examination boards in the UK

Examination boards in the UK that grant professional qualifications in advanced techniques of epilation are:

The Institute of Electrolysis
Emsdene
Church Street
Warwickshire CV35 9LS
Tel: 01789 471571   Fax: 0870 081 3611
Email: institute@electrolysis.co.uk

The British Association of Electrolysists Ltd
40 Parkfield Road
Ickenham
Uxbridge
Middlesex
Tel: 0870 1280477 Fax: 0870 1330407
Email: sec@baeltd.fsbusiness.co.uk

The Confederation of International Beauty Therapy and Cosmetology
BABTAC Office
70 Eastgate Street
Gloucester GL1 1QN
Tel: 01452 421114 Fax: 01452 421110
Email: lorraine@babtac.com

EDEXCEL
Stuart House
Russell Square
London WC1B 5DN

City & Guilds
76 Portland Place
London W1N 4AA
Tel: 0207 1278 2468

Vocational Training Charitable Trust
46 Aldwich Road
Bognor Reigis
West Sussex PO21 2PN
Tel: 01243 842064

International Therapy Examination Centre (ITEC)
4 Heathfield Terrace
Chiswick
London W4 4JE
Tel: 0208 994 4141 Fax: 0208 994 7880

Index

Page numbers in **bold** refer to illustrations

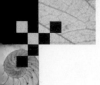

Index

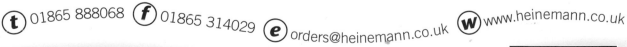
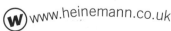
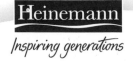